FULL-BODY
flexibility

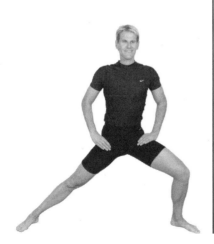

FULL-BODY
flexibility

Jay Blahnik

Human Kinetics

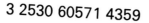

3 2530 60571 4359

Library of Congress Cataloging-in-Publication Data

Blahnik, Jay.
 Full-body flexibility / Jay Blahnik.
    p. cm.
 Includes index.
  ISBN 0-7360-4150-8 (Soft cover)
  1. Stretching exercises. I. Title: Full body flexibility. II. Title.
 RA781.63.B56 2004
 613.7'182--dc22

                    2003017849

ISBN: 0-7360-4150-8

Acquisitions Editor: Martin Barnard; **Developmental Editor:** Laura Hambly; **Assistant Editors:** Alisha Jeddeloh, Anna FitzSimmons, and Kim Thoren; **Copyeditor:** John Wentworth; **Proofreader:** Myla Smith; **Indexer:** Bobbi Swanson; **Graphic Designer:** Nancy Rasmus; **Graphic Artist:** Denise Lowry; **Art and Photo Manager:** Dan Wendt; **Cover Designer:** Keith Blomberg; **Photographer (cover and interior):** Stephen Ryan Photographics; **Illustrator:** Argosy Publishing; **Printer:** Bang Printing

Human Kinetics books are available at special discounts for bulk purchase. Special editions or book excerpts can also be created to specification. For details, contact the Special Sales Manager at Human Kinetics.

Printed in the United States of America   10   9   8   7   6   5   4   3   2   1

Human Kinetics
Web site: www.HumanKinetics.com

United States: Human Kinetics, P.O. Box 5076, Champaign, IL 61825-5076
800-747-4457
e-mail: humank@hkusa.com

Canada: Human Kinetics, 475 Devonshire Road Unit 100, Windsor, ON N8Y 2L5
800-465-7301 (in Canada only)
e-mail: orders@hkcanada.com

Europe: Human Kinetics, 107 Bradford Road, Stanningley, Leeds LS28 6AT, United Kingdom
+44 (0) 113 255 5665
e-mail: hk@hkeurope.com

Australia: Human Kinetics, 57A Price Avenue, Lower Mitcham, South Australia 5062
08 8277 1555
e-mail: liaw@hkaustralia.com

New Zealand: Human Kinetics, Division of Sports Distributors NZ Ltd.
P.O. Box 300 226 Albany, North Shore City, Auckland
0064 9 448 1207
e-mail: blairc@hknewz.com

This book is dedicated to my parents,
David and Charlene Blahnik.

You taught me that hard work, a good attitude,
and the belief that anything is possible
are the only tools you need to be successful.

I love you with all my heart.

Part I   Total Body Stretch System

CONTENTS

PREFACE

You probably picked up this book because you have an active lifestyle, you enjoy working out or playing sports, and you know that you should stretch more. It feels good to stretch, and the research indicates it's smart to stretch. So why does stretching always seem to take the back seat to other exercise activities?

I have been training and coaching fitness enthusiasts and athletes for almost 20 years, and I think I know the answer. I believe people generally don't stretch enough because the benefits and results of traditional stretching are difficult to measure. Too often, people simply do a few of the stretches they remember from P.E. class before or after they work out. But many of those traditional stretches don't necessarily provide the right balance of stretches your body needs. Therefore, people don't necessarily provide the right balance of stretches your body needs. Therefore, people don't see and feel the results they are looking for. And even if you are doing *some* effective stretches, most people (including many athletes and fitness authorities) don't know how to put together a *whole* stretch routine that gets results.

Full-Body Flexibility can change that. The three-step stretch system I've developed for this book gives you a unique but simple system for stretching that will improve your flexibility, mobility, and strength in a way you can see, feel, and truly benefit from. Once you have learned and are ready to take advantage of the three-step system, you'll find more than 100 stretches to help you target the areas that need stretching most. The 13 enjoyable stretch routines in part II make it easy and fun to stretch anywhere, anytime. Whether you're searching to improve your overall fitness or sport performance or just looking for a more effective way to stretch, *Full-Body Flexibility* gives you the right tools to reduce the tension in your muscles, make you stronger, lubricate your joints, refresh your body, make it easier to reach and bend for things, make you a better athlete, and help you stand taller.

Considering how much this book promises to deliver, you might expect the content to be complicated, flashy, or hard to do. But it isn't any of those things. In fact, this is a great book for beginners as well as serious athletes and the very fit. I use the system and the routines in this book myself and have taught hundreds of other trainers, fitness instructors, and coaches how to use them to aid their clients and athletes in their pursuit of greater flexibility and overall fitness. The system and the routines can work for nearly anyone, and the photos and clear instructions make it easy to get started right away.

This book is divided into two parts. Part I includes more than 100 stretches that work your body from head to toe. Part I is also your reference guide for the routines in part II. Until you learn the stretches well, refer to part I for clear instructions on how to perform all the stretches you want to do. I have divided the body into four regions, each with its own chapter, to make it easy to locate a muscle group or stretch and to understand the benefits of doing the stretches. For example, chapter 2 contains stretches for the neck, shoulders, arms, and hands. These stretches reduce tension and play a part in preventing common occupational ailments such as carpal tunnel syndrome. Chapter 3 includes stretches for the chest, back, and abdominals. The stretches lengthen and strengthen these muscles, helping to improve posture and alleviate back pain.

Part II introduces you to several stretch routines that use the same stretches you have learned in part I. Part II contains fitness routines and sports routines as well as specialty stretch routines.

In the fitness routines, the stretches are organized in a way that makes it quick and easy for you to get a good stretch workout. The fitness routines are divided into 10-, 20-, and 40-minute routines, so there's always one to choose no matter how much time you have.

The sports routines show you the proper performance and recovery stretches for dozens of different sports. For example, the routine for cyclists focuses on alleviating tight shoulders and sore quadriceps, whereas the routine for basketball helps you jump higher and reach farther. The sports are divided into three categories by type of movement, which helps you easily find your favorite sports.

The specialty stretch routines in chapter 9 let you focus on one area of the body or stretch with a goal in mind. For example, one stretch routine helps wake you up in the morning; another helps you relax before going to sleep at night. One routine helps with lower back problems, another with tight shoulders and neck. I suggest many ways to fit stretching into your everyday life comfortably, quickly, and easily.

You can pick up dozens of books on stretching, and each one might endorse a slightly different approach or philosophy on how to go about it. What method do you choose? What method is the safest? And how am I so sure *this* book will give you the greatest results? As a fitness veteran, I'm savvy enough not to claim to have the last word on stretching. There is always something new to learn, which is part of what makes exercise fun. However, there are stretching techniques and ideas that most experts agree are effective. The problem up to now was that these great techniques were never compiled in a single book with all the routines you need to succeed. Now that book is here. In *Full-Body Flexibility*, I offer you the best stretches and stretch routines within a practical system that will change what stretching can do for you.

ACKNOWLEDGMENTS

Although I work full-time in the health and fitness industry and I have dedicated my life to educating people about proper exercise, writing a book about it was not easy for me. Not just because of my travel schedule, but also because anyone who knows me can attest to the fact that I am a speaker at heart, not a writer. Because of this, completing this book required a great deal of help from a number of people whom I would like to thank.

Martin Barnard, senior acquisitions editor at Human Kinetics, brought this amazing opportunity to me a number of years ago. It is because of him that this book was written. He was patient when I missed my deadlines, supportive of the direction I wanted to take, and provided tremendous clarity to me as the book unfolded. He is a first-class human being, and I cannot thank him enough for everything he did to bring *Full-Body Flexibility* to life.

Laura Hambly, my editor at Human Kinetics, somehow managed to edit my work and boost my self-esteem at the same time! She was incredibly helpful at taking what I provided and giving it the extra sense of clarity that made it so much better than it otherwise would have been. I would also like to thank her and designer Nancy Rasmus for creating the incredible design that makes this book so easy to follow and user-friendly.

Phil and Juliane Arney and Julie LaFond, my best friends and business partners, provided research, edited my ideas, and were always there to brainstorm and give direction. In addition, they both allowed me to bounce ideas off them and test my routines time and time again. I could not have completed this project without their help.

Ben Rubin, MD, the most talented doctor, surgeon, and health professional I know, has helped me through multiple strains, pains, and injuries throughout my career. He has also provided me with world-class advice and exercise information that has helped me beyond measure. Most importantly, Ben has inspired me to be the best professional I can be.

Steve Ryan was the photographer for this book. He is talented and kind, and I appreciate his hard work and contribution.

Kate Katke, Maria Hamilton, and Juliane Arney were the models that made the photos look so incredibly beautiful by lending us their gorgeous faces and bodies. Thank you for being involved with this project.

It is impossible to fully express the gratitude I feel toward these people who have helped me complete this book, but my heart is as grateful as it can be.

PART I

Total Body
Stretch System

CHAPTER 1

Preparing to Stretch

Neck, Shoulders, Arms, and Hands

Chest, Back, and Abdominals

Buttocks, Hips, Quadriceps, and Hamstrings

Calves, Shins, and Feet

Multiregion Stretches

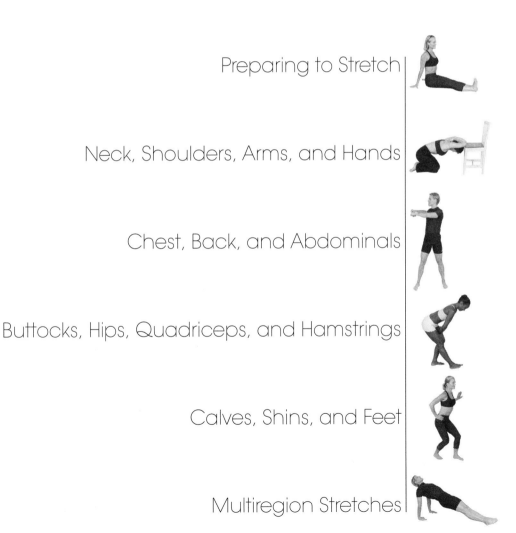

Preparing to Stretch

If you're like me, you're anxious to get going and would rather skip the reading and jump right into a few stretches. But before you dive in, take a deep breath and read this chapter. It won't take long. You'll come out of it with a clear understanding of the stretch system we use in the book and of how to maximize the benefits of the information, graphics, and photos. You'll probably have to read this chapter just once, and it's worth it!

STRETCHING TECHNIQUES

First we'll review a few important stretching techniques and terms you should understand before you begin. Even if you're very familiar with stretching, it's a good idea to double-check your knowledge of this information. Believe it or not, even personal trainers and exercise specialists get confused and misuse these terms and their applications.

Assisted and Unassisted Stretching

Also known in the scientific world as *passive stretching,* assisted stretching simply means that you're using some sort of outside assistance to help you achieve a stretch. This assistance could be your body weight, a strap, leverage, or even gravity. With assisted stretching, you relax the muscle you're trying to stretch and rely on the external force to hold you in place. Assisted stretching is the most common form of stretching because it's easy to do and generally the most comfortable. You don't usually have to work very hard to do an assisted stretch, but there's always the risk that the external force will be stronger than you are flexible, which could cause an injury. You need to be mindful and aware of that, and you need to use good technique. Assisted stretches are most commonly used to increase flexibility.

However, because you don't have to use your own muscle strength to initiate the stretch, assisted stretching has come to be considered less helpful for improving movement in everyday life or in sport performance. In other words, you might improve your flexibility if you do only assisted stretching, but you might not improve your active range of motion for jumping, running, playing, walking, and reaching.

Unassisted stretching, also known as *active stretching*, simply means that you're stretching one muscle by actively contracting another one, usually the muscle in opposition to the one you're stretching. With unassisted stretching, you don't use assistance, leverage, or gravity to help you with the stretch. For example, squeezing your shoulder blades together and contracting your back muscles is an example of an unassisted chest stretch. Unassisted stretching is much less common and less popular than assisted stretching because it takes more effort and can be difficult to do. However, unassisted stretching has come to be considered very helpful for improving movement in everyday life and sport performance because it requires you to use and build your own strength while you improve your flexibility. Unassisted stretches can also be helpful in improving your posture because they often require you to work the muscles in your back and abdominals (known as your core or trunk power center). So, along with easing your everyday movements, incorporating unassisted stretching into your routine might provide bonus benefits.

Static and Dynamic Stretching

Whether you're doing an assisted stretch or an unassisted stretch, you can choose to hold the stretch (static) or keep the stretch in motion (dynamic). When you do a stretch statically, you should generally hold the position somewhere between 10 and 30 seconds. When you stretch dynamically, you should move through the stretch 10 or 12 times. Although static stretching is more common, dynamic stretching has incredible benefits and has recently been associated with improved sport performance and enhanced everyday mobility.

One warning: Don't confuse dynamic stretching with old-fashioned ballistic stretching (remember the bouncing toe touches from PE class?). Dynamic stretching is controlled, smooth, and deliberate. Ballistic stretching is jerky, uncontrolled, and erratic. Ballistic stretching can damage muscles and joints and should be avoided except under the supervision of a professional. For most people, the risks of ballistic stretching far outweigh the benefits.

The calf stretches on page 5 illustrate assisted, unassisted, static, and dynamic stretches.

There are lots of fancy techniques used in stretching (especially by coaches and athletes), such as PNF (proprioceptive neuromuscular facilitation) stretching or AI (active isolated) stretching. However, these techniques are still either assisted or unassisted stretches and are executed either statically

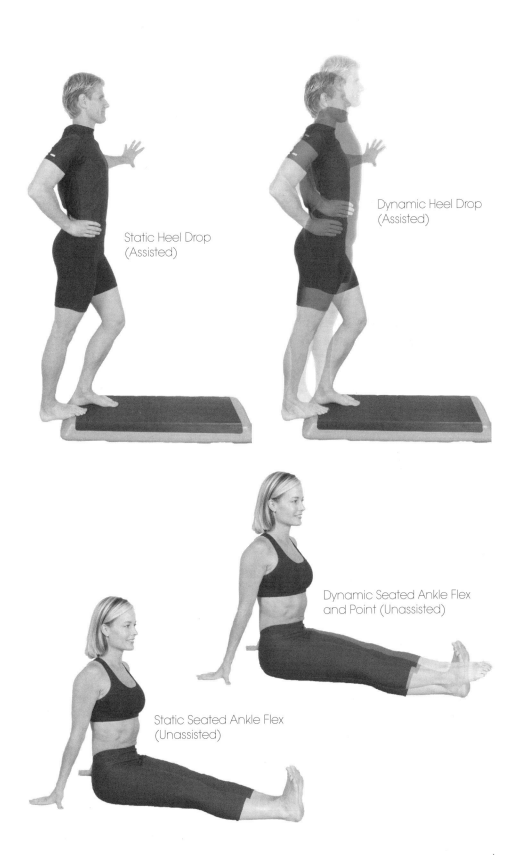

Static Heel Drop
(Assisted)

Dynamic Heel Drop
(Assisted)

Dynamic Seated Ankle Flex
and Point (Unassisted)

Static Seated Ankle Flex
(Unassisted)

or dynamically. The fancy variations are simply techniques used to speed up the process of achieving flexibility (often at some risk to the person doing the technique) or to enhance range of motion beyond the point required for most people. Don't get me wrong—I use many of these techniques with my clients and students as well, but most are too complex to do correctly without an instructor, trainer, or coach. And, at the end of the day, they are simply variations of one of these four stretching techniques.

STRETCHING EFFECTIVELY

Whenever I teach a stretch to a client or student, I expect to be asked these questions:

> Where should I feel the stretch?
>
> Am I doing the stretch correctly and safely?
>
> How do I make the stretch more (or less) challenging?

Because the human body is so complex, subtle shifts in body weight, position, and direction of movement can greatly affect how a stretch feels, whether it's safe or not, and how challenging it is. Because these three questions are so basic, I want to answer each of them for every stretch in the book. For convenience, this book includes both written instructions and visual cues for each stretch so that you can read and see what you're supposed to be doing. In addition, I want you to know how your flexibility measures up to the norm so you'll be able to direct your focus to the areas of your body that most need to be stretched.

The following is a breakdown of how to review each stretch in the book.

Assisted or unassisted—For each muscle group, you'll find several stretches. The assisted stretches bear the label "assisted stretch" down the side of the page, and the unassisted stretches are indicated with the words "unassisted stretch."

Stretch descriptions—Each stretch includes simple written instructions for execution. This is also where you'll see whether the stretch is static or dynamic. Because dynamic stretching involves movement, there will generally be instructions and photos for starting and finishing the movement as well as a reminder of how many repetitions to do.

Targeted muscle groups—You'll want to know which muscle group you're targeting for each stretch you do. In each stretch description, I have listed the muscles indicating where you should feel the stretch. If necessary, you can refer to the anatomy diagrams on pages 12-13 to see where these muscles are. This should help you adjust your positioning for each stretch to ensure you're targeting the right muscle group.

Range of motion—Each photo shows a person with an ideal range of motion for a particular stretch. Think of range of motion in three categories:

1. Tight—below average range of motion
2. Ideal—normal range of motion
3. Extraordinary—exceptional range of motion

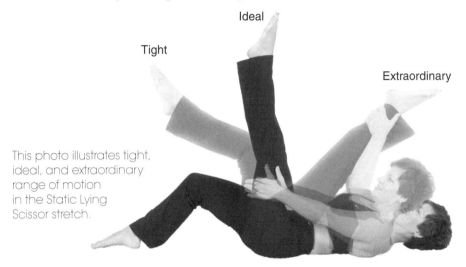

This photo illustrates tight, ideal, and extraordinary range of motion in the Static Lying Scissor stretch.

If you can perform a stretch with the same technique and execution as shown in the photo, you likely have ideal range of motion for that stretch. If you're unable to get into the stretch as shown in the photo, you're likely tight for that stretch. If you're able to move farther in the direction of the stretch (with good technique), you likely have extraordinary range of motion for that stretch.

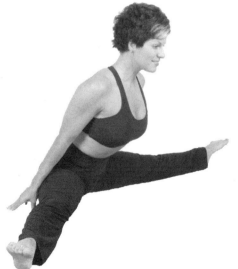

It is very important that you move deeper into a stretch only if you are comfortably able to move in the correct direction with *good technique*. For example, if you are able to move your rib cage forward, *but only by rounding your shoulders*, you should not take the stretch any farther.

WHEN TO STRETCH

Although stretching before a workout has long been recommended as an effective way to reduce the risk of injury, there has been a great deal of controversy surrounding this subject in recent years. Believe it or not, some of the current research suggests that fit people who stretch before they work out actually have a *higher* rate of injury than those who don't.

This might seem puzzling, but when you think further, the reasons become clear. Although stretching on a regular basis can provide a host of wonderful benefits (including increased flexibility), the actual act of stretching can be quite stressful on the muscles and joints. When we stretch a muscle, we're causing microscopic damage to soft tissue that ultimately repairs itself, which can lead to greater mobility. However, in the minutes immediately following stretching, the soft tissue is in a state of stress, which makes it more difficult for the muscle to produce the power and force usually required in a workout activity or sport.

For example, if you stretch before you go for a run, you might very well be making it more difficult for your muscles to generate the power and force required of your body during the run. And the normal stress of the run combined with the stress from the pre-exercise stretches can put the body at greater risk than if you did not stretch at all before the run.

It is interesting, however, that the research also seems to indicate that a good warm-up can in fact reduce the risk of injury prior to a workout *if* the warm-up is designed appropriately for the workout that follows. For example, a five- to eight-minute power walk or easy jog before a run at normal running pace likely reduces the risk of injury during the run. A few knee-lift hugs, small kicks, small jumps, shoulder rolls, side steps, and some light running would probably be an effective warm-up for a soccer game.

Based on the research, the best time to stretch is either *after* a workout, when the soft tissues are warm and pliable, or as a *stand-alone* workout that won't be followed by anything powerful or intense. For example, you can stretch at your desk for as little as five minutes or at the end of the day for as long as 30 minutes. You can stretch after a vigorous weight-training workout or soccer game. But you shouldn't stretch *before* your weight-training workout or soccer game. Instead, warm up lightly in a way that gently introduces your muscles to the upcoming activity, and save your stretching for after the activity is over.

I know that many of you reading this have been stretching before your workout for years, and what I'm saying might be a bit of a shock. In my experience, people who stretch before they work out are attached to doing it that way and very reluctant to change. In fact, many of my clients and athletes insist they absolutely *do* find that pre-exercise stretching helps with their performance, range of motion, and power when they work out or play a sport.

It's hard to argue with what feels right for any particular person. So, take what I'm saying to heart (because the research is persuasive), but if you *do* stretch before you exercise, that doesn't mean you're automatically going to get injured. In fact, it might not harm your performance at all. Just remember that there's no indication that stretching will *help* your performance or reduce your risk of injury if you do it before you work out or play a sport.

If you choose to do the stretches or routines in this book before you work out, please go easy—don't be overaggressive if you're planning to work out or play a sport immediately afterward. Listen to your body and do what feels right for you.

THREE-STEP STRETCH SYSTEM

This book probably includes more stretches than you'll ever need. Even so, you must approach your stretching in a specific way if you want optimal success. Whether your goal is to increase your flexibility, get through your day more easily, or improve your performance on the athletic field, you should have a plan.

Over the years, I have come up with a stretch system that works incredibly well in my classes and with my clients. This system includes just three simple steps to focus on when stretching: *variety, strength,* and *balance.*

> Step 1: Variety. Your stretch routines should contain both assisted and unassisted stretches.
>
> Step 2: Strength. Use unassisted stretches to build strength that supports your flexibility.
>
> Step 3: Balance. Work toward balance in the right and left and in the front and back sides of your body.

Variety

In the routines in part II, I have tried to make it easy for you to balance assisted and unassisted stretches in your regimen by including both. However, as you progress in your stretching program, you'll likely begin making up your own routines or focusing on muscle groups that are particularly tight for you. When you do this, just remember not to spend all your time on assisted stretches. Because there are many more assisted stretches than there are unassisted, it's easy to neglect the unassisted stretches—but don't. You'll find the benefits are greater when you include both types. An easy way to make *variety* a habit is to do the two types of stretches back to back. For example, do the Dynamic Heel Drop followed by the Static Seated Ankle Flex.

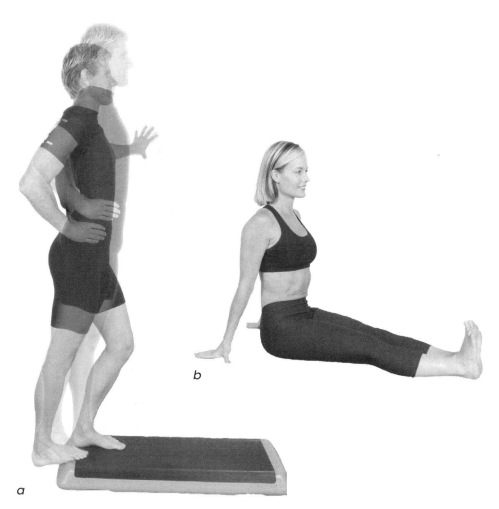

Vary your routine by doing assisted and unassisted stretches back to back, as in (a) the Dynamic Heel Drop and (b) the Static Seated Ankle Flex.

Strength

Use unassisted stretches to build *strength* that supports your flexibility. This involves getting as good at the unassisted stretches as you are at the assisted stretches. For example, if you have ideal or extraordinary range of motion when you execute the Static Lying Scissor stretch, but you struggle with the Dynamic Lying Scissor stretch (both stretch the hamstring group), you're likely not as strong as you are flexible. Play to your weakness and be slightly more aggressive when you do the Dynamic Lying Scissor stretch. This helps your flexibility and strength remain in balance—you don't become too flexible without the strength to support the flexibility. This doesn't mean you should stop doing the assisted stretch you're so good at. Go ahead and do it, but don't push yourself farther until your unassisted stretch comes closer to matching it.

Balance

Pay attention to your body's muscular imbalances and work to improve them. For example, if you notice your right hip is tighter than your left hip, be a little more aggressive when you stretch the right hip until you feel the hips have a similar range of motion. Don't be surprised if you notice many subtle imbalances when you're stretching. I notice them all the time when I'm stretching. It's normal and gives you something to work on!

Also try to be aware of how the muscles on the front side of one area of your body compare to the muscles on the reverse side of the same area of your body. For example, you might notice that you have ideal or extraordinary flexibility in your quadriceps but that you're quite tight in your hamstrings (very common). If so, spend more time on your hamstring stretches than on your quadriceps stretches until you feel these muscles are closer to being equally flexible.

It's important to incorporate the three-step system when stretching. Maybe you're asking, "Why can't I just do the stretches? Won't that be good enough?" The truth is you *can* just stretch without paying attention to the three steps. If you're not stretching at all now, then yes, just doing some stretches is an improvement. But over the years we've seen a higher rate of injuries in athletes (and non-athletes, too) who don't focus on *variety, strength,* and *balance* when they stretch. In fact, we've found that many people who frequently stretch still injure themselves when they could have prevented it by incorporating these three simple steps.

For example, runners often develop lower-leg injuries (shin splints) because their calves are tighter than their shins are strong. Stretches incorporating strength can help with this problem because they focus on strengthening the shin and stretching the calves using a variety of unassisted calf stretches.

Poor posture (one of the leading causes of chronic back pain) is often caused by our spending all day using our chest and shoulders to move our arms across the *front* of the body but rarely using our back muscles to pull the arms *behind* the body. Consequently, we get tight chest muscles and overly flexible back muscles. Stretching with balance in mind would help with this problem because you'd be spending more time stretching your chest than stretching your back, which helps improve your posture.

If you stretch regularly, you'll probably become more flexible, but if you stretch regularly using the *variety, strength,* and *balance* system of stretching, you'll likely see a list of benefits that far exceeds just increased flexibility. Stretching alone is good for you, but stretching using the three-step system is great for you. The system is one of the key components of this book and will make your stretching experience and results rewarding.

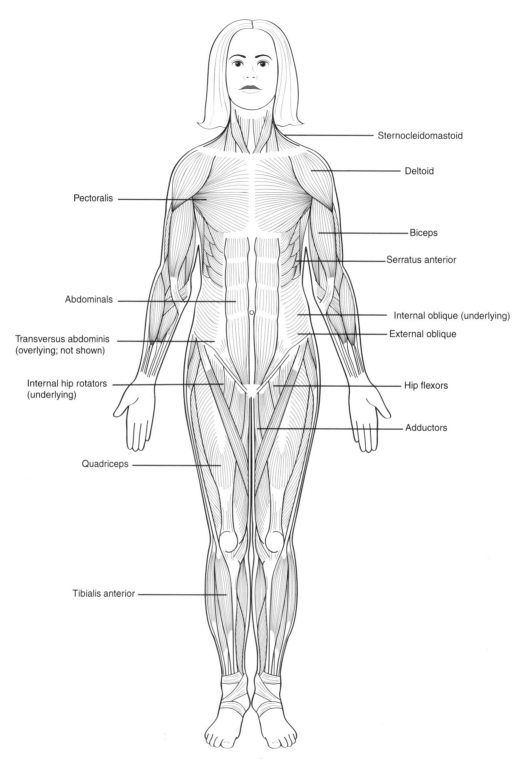

- Sternocleidomastoid
- Deltoid
- Pectoralis
- Biceps
- Serratus anterior
- Abdominals
- Internal oblique (underlying)
- External oblique
- Transversus abdominis (overlying; not shown)
- Internal hip rotators (underlying)
- Hip flexors
- Adductors
- Quadriceps
- Tibialis anterior

Full-body muscle diagram. Use this diagram to identify targeted muscle groups.

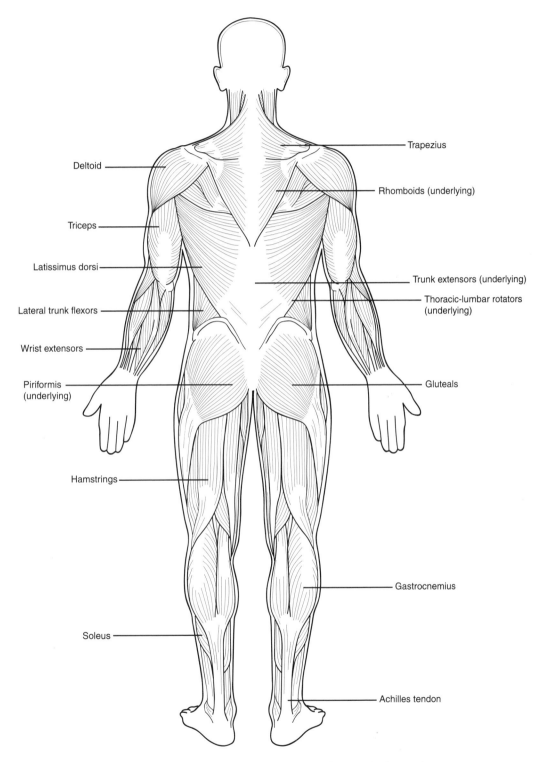

Trapezius

Deltoid

Rhomboids (underlying)

Triceps

Latissimus dorsi

Trunk extensors (underlying)

Thoracic-lumbar rotators (underlying)

Lateral trunk flexors

Wrist extensors

Piriformis (underlying)

Gluteals

Hamstrings

Gastrocnemius

Soleus

Achilles tendon

Full-body muscle diagram. Use this diagram to identify targeted muscle groups.

CHAPTER 2

Neck, Shoulders, Arms, and Hands

In this chapter we'll focus on stretching the muscles that support the head and control the movement of the arms and hands. Don't be surprised to find yourself tighter than you might expect with some of these stretches. These muscles tend to be overlooked in most people's flexibility routines, even though they're as important as all the other muscle groups for total body function and power.

Remember that the photos and graphics are designed to guide you through each stretch safely and effectively. Also recall that the person in each photo is representing the ideal range of motion for that particular stretch. Take your time with each stretch, and don't force anything. Each person is different. Your body will be ready for some stretches and not so ready for others. This gives you the opportunity to mark your body's adjustments and really feel the results!

NECK

I think you'll be pleasantly surprised how relaxing and rewarding it is to do the neck stretches. These stretches help with many daily tasks we take for granted, such as looking over your shoulder to change lanes on the freeway or looking up to catch a ball or watch an airplane.

Static Head Tilt

Sternocleidomastoid, trapezius

Stand or sit tall. Lower one ear toward the shoulder. Gently pull down from the opposite side of the head.

Hold the stretch for 10 to 30 seconds.

Repeat on the other side.

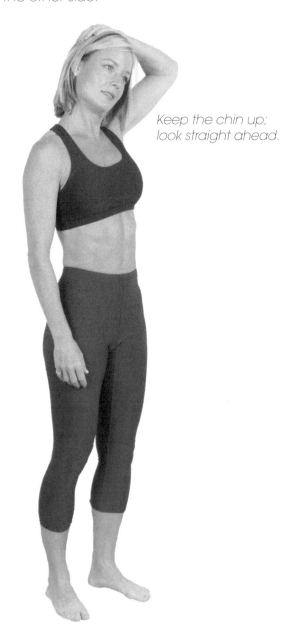

Keep the chin up; look straight ahead.

ASSISTED STRETCH

16

Static Diagonal Head Tilt

Sternocleidomastoid, trapezius

Stand or sit tall. Drop the chin diagonally toward the armpit as far as comfortably possible. Place one hand on the back of the head and gently pull toward the armpit.

Hold the stretch for 10 to 30 seconds.

Repeat on the other side.

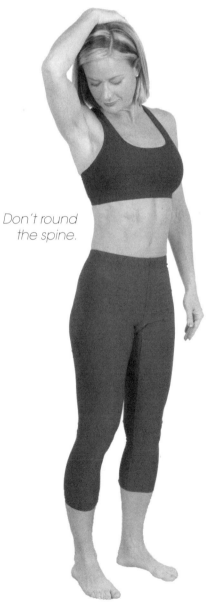

Don't round the spine.

Static Head Turn

Sternocleidomastoid, trapezius

Stand or sit tall.

Turn the head as far to one side as comfortably possible. Place one hand on the side of the chin and gently push.

Hold the stretch for 10 to 30 seconds.

Repeat on the other side.

Keep the chin up.

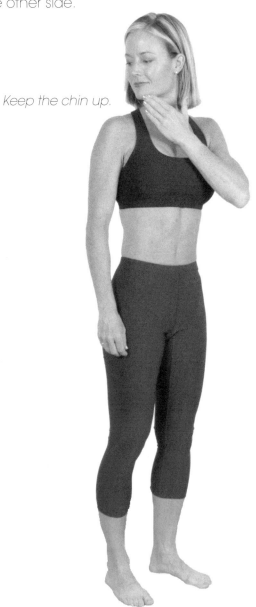

Dynamic Head Tilt

Sternocleidomastoid, trapezius

Stand or sit tall.

Start: Lower one ear toward the shoulder while lifting the opposite ear toward the ceiling.

Finish: Release the stretch and repeat on the other side.

Repeat as a continuous, controlled, fluid sequence 10 to 12 times.

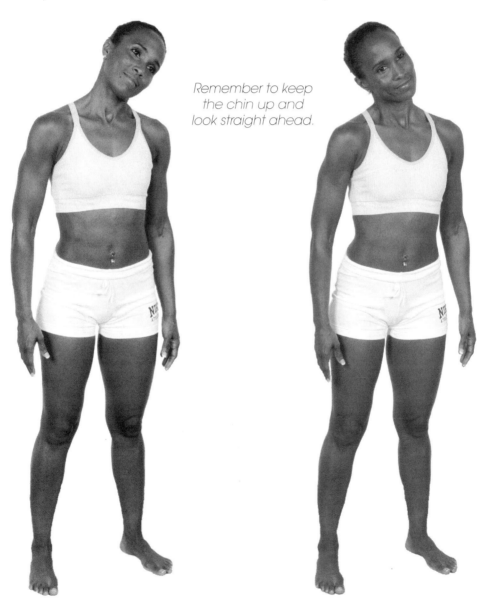

Remember to keep the chin up and look straight ahead.

Dynamic Head Turn

Sternocleidomastoid, trapezius

Stand or sit tall.

Start: Turn the head as far to one side as comfortably possible.

Finish: Release the stretch and turn the head to the other side.

Keep the chin up.

Repeat as a continuous, controlled, fluid sequence 10 to 12 times.

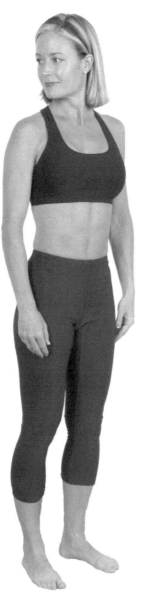
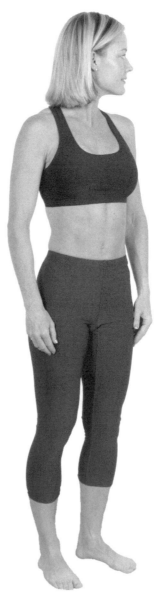

Dynamic Diagonal Chin Drop

Sternocleidomastoid, trapezius

Stand or sit tall.

Start: Drop the chin diagonally toward the armpit as far as comfortably possible while lifting the back of the head toward the ceiling.

Finish: Release the stretch by lifting the head to neutral position and repeat on the other side.

Repeat as a continuous, controlled, fluid sequence 10 to 12 times.

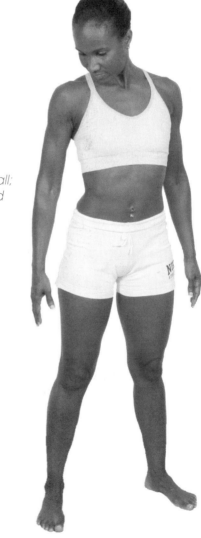

Stand or sit tall; don't round the spine.

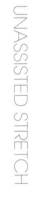

SHOULDERS

The muscles that control the movement of the shoulders are the trapezius (the kite-shaped muscle on the back) and the deltoids, which cover the front, top, and rear of the shoulder joint. Stretching these muscles improves your posture and makes it easier to reach up or behind you.

Static Reach-Behind Head Tilt

Trapezius

Stand with the feet apart and the arms next to the body. Slowly drop the head to one side. Reach behind and pull down on the wrist of the opposite arm.

Hold the stretch for 10 to 30 seconds.

Repeat on the other side.

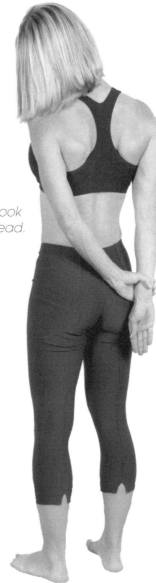

Stand tall; look straight ahead.

Static Seated Head Tilt

Trapezius

Sit with the legs in front of the body and the knees slightly bent. Reach out as far as possible to both sides, touching the floor; slowly drop the head to one side.

Hold the stretch for 10 to 30 seconds.

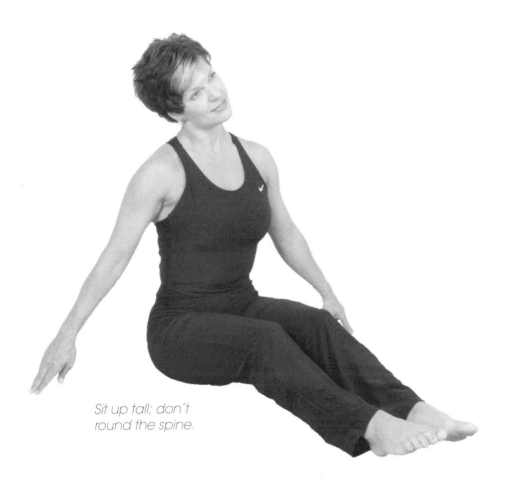

Sit up tall; don't round the spine.

Dynamic Chin Drop

Trapezius

Stand with the feet apart and arms alongside the body.

Start: Slowly drop the head forward and gently bring the chin closer to the chest.

Finish: Release the stretch by lifting the head to a neutral position.

Repeat as a continuous, controlled, fluid sequence 10 to 12 times.

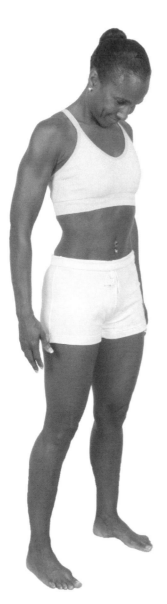

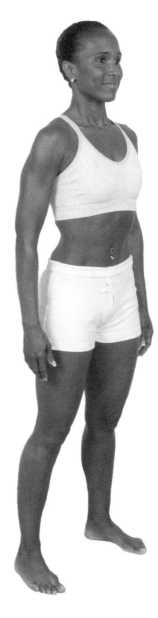

Stand tall; don't round the spine.

Static Flyaway

Deltoid (front shoulder)

Stand with the feet apart. Lift the arms out to the side of the body at shoulder height, palms facing down. Reach behind as far as comfortably possible.

Hold the stretch for 10 to 30 seconds.

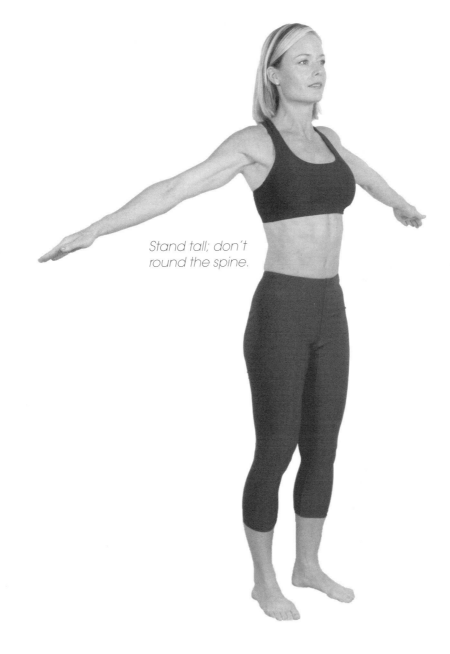

Stand tall; don't round the spine.

Static Behind and Open

Deltoid (front shoulder)

Stand with the feet shoulder-width apart. Clasp the hands together in the small of the back and lift the arms upward.

Hold the stretch for 10 to 30 seconds.

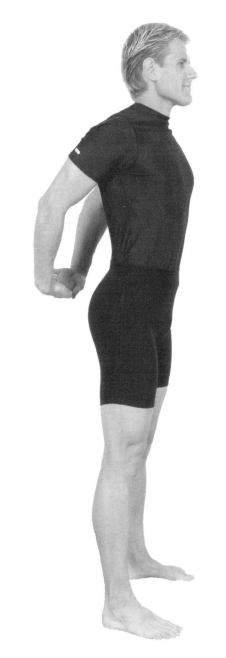

Stand tall; don't round the spine.

Dynamic Flyaway

Deltoid (front shoulder)

Stand with feet apart.

Start: Lift arms a few inches away from the hips; slowly lift the arms behind the body.

Finish: Release the stretch by returning the arms to the side of the body.

Repeat as a continuous, controlled, fluid sequence 10 to 12 times.

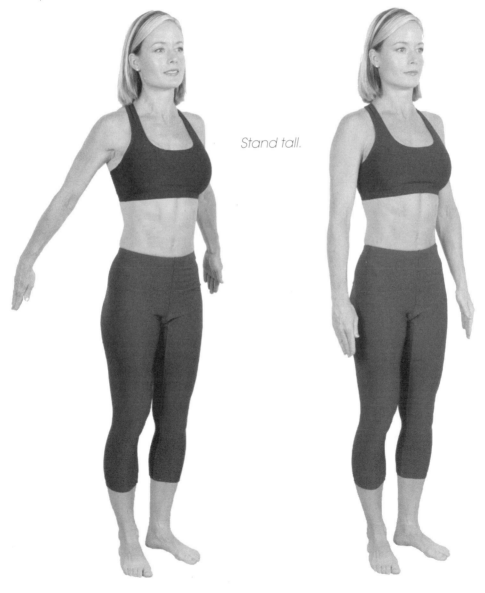

Stand tall.

Dynamic Kneeling Shoulder Push

Deltoid (front shoulder)

Kneel on the floor on the hands and knees.

Start: Gently push one shoulder toward the floor.

Finish: Release stretch by moving the shoulder level with the opposite shoulder.

Repeat on the other side.

Repeat as a continuous, controlled, fluid sequence 10 to 12 times.

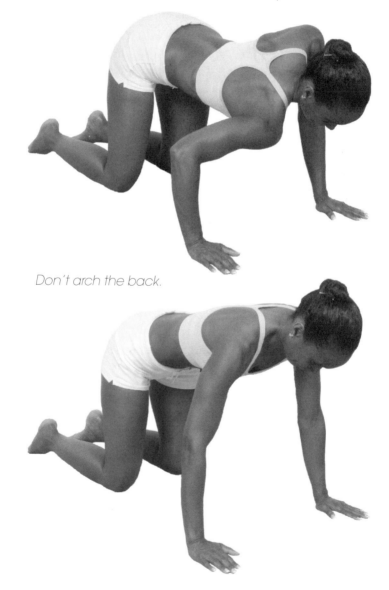

Don't arch the back.

Dynamic Seated Shoulder Push

Deltoid (front shoulder)

Sit down; place both legs straight in front with knees slightly bent.

Start: Place the hands behind the body and press one shoulder toward the feet.

Finish: Release the stretch by moving the shoulder level with the opposite shoulder. Repeat on the other side.

Repeat as a continuous, controlled, fluid sequence 10 to 12 times.

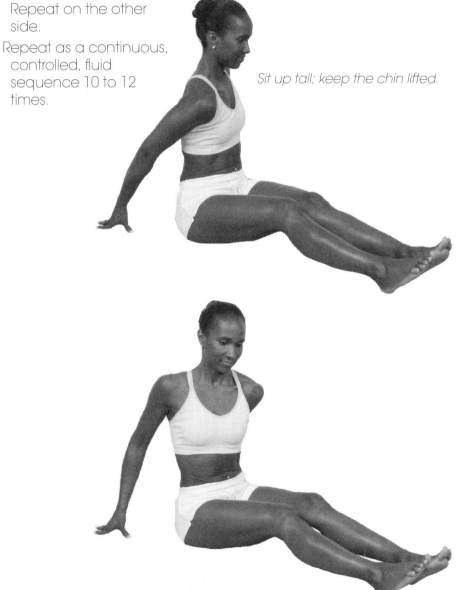

Sit up tall; keep the chin lifted.

Dynamic Faucet Hands

Deltoid (front shoulder)

Stand with the arms in front of the body at shoulder height, palms facing each other.

Start: Twist the hands inward as far as possible (similar to turning faucets).

Finish: Twist the hands in the opposite direction.

Repeat as a continuous, controlled, fluid sequence 10 to 12 times.

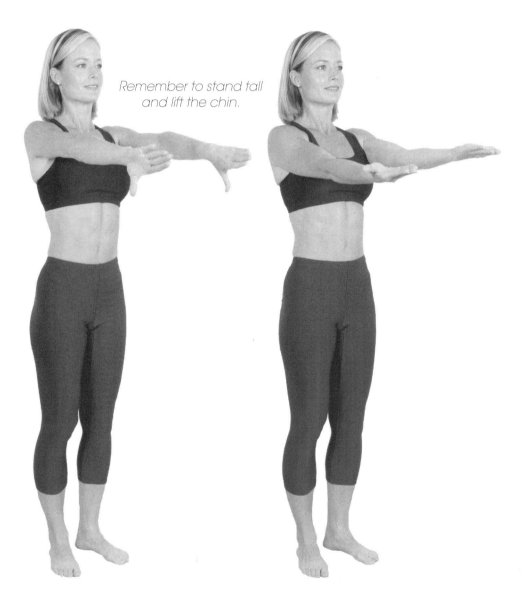

Remember to stand tall and lift the chin.

Static Straight Arm Across

Deltoid (rear shoulder)

Stand with feet shoulder-width apart. Bring one arm across the body at chest height and hold it in place with the opposite arm.

Hold the stretch for 10 to 30 seconds.

Repeat on the other arm.

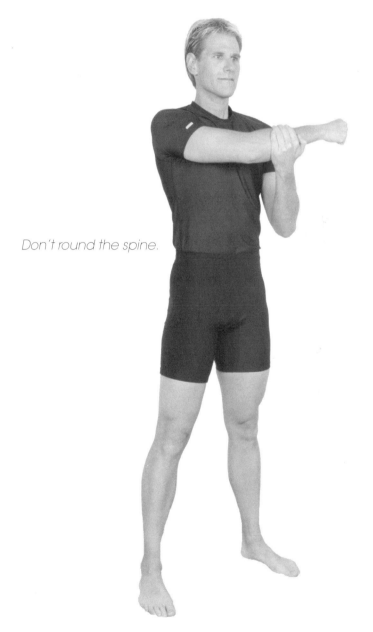

Don't round the spine.

Dynamic Arm Across

Deltoid (rear shoulder)

Stand with feet apart.

Start: Bring one arm across the body at chest height as far as comfortably possible.

Finish: Release the stretch by bringing the arm out to the side of the body at chest height.

Repeat as a continuous, controlled, fluid sequence 10 to 12 times.

Repeat on the other arm.

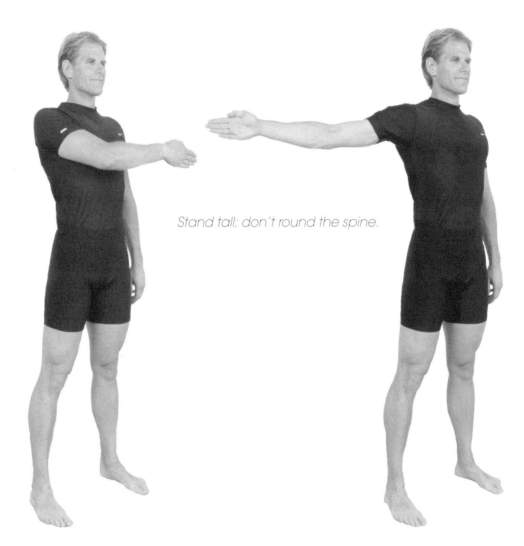

Stand tall; don't round the spine.

Dynamic Shoulder Push

Deltoid (rear shoulder)

Stand with feet shoulder-width apart and arms lifted to shoulder height.

Start: Roll one shoulder toward the feet.

Finish: Release the stretch by rolling the shoulder back to a neutral position.

Repeat as a continuous, controlled, fluid sequence 10 to 12 times on both sides of the body.

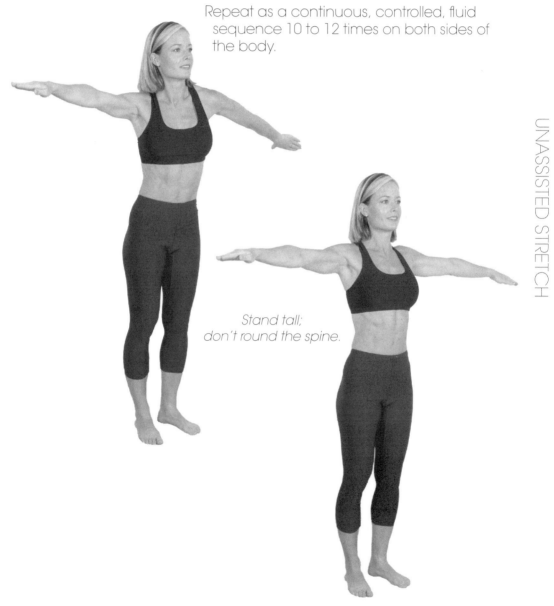

Stand tall; don't round the spine.

ARMS

We're pushing, pulling, lifting, and lowering things all day long. Improved mobility in the arms helps make these tasks easier.

Static Pronated Reach-Back and Turn

Biceps

Stand and raise the arm out to the side at shoulder height. Place the back of the hand (thumb down) against a stationary object, such as a wall or door. Slowly rotate the upper body away from the hand.

Hold the stretch for 10 to 30 seconds.

Repeat on the other arm.

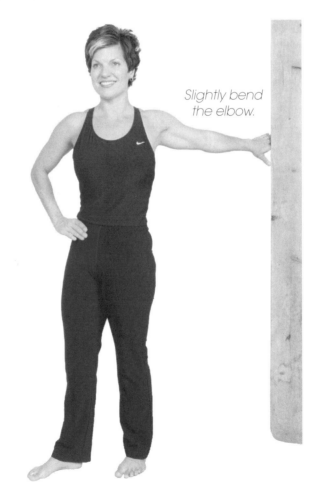

Slightly bend the elbow.

Dynamic Rotated Flyaway

Biceps

Stand tall with hands at the sides and palms facing back.

Start: Lift arms behind the body and toward the ceiling while twisting palms outward.

Finish: Release the stretch by returning to setup position.

Repeat as a continuous, controlled, fluid sequence 10 to 12 times.

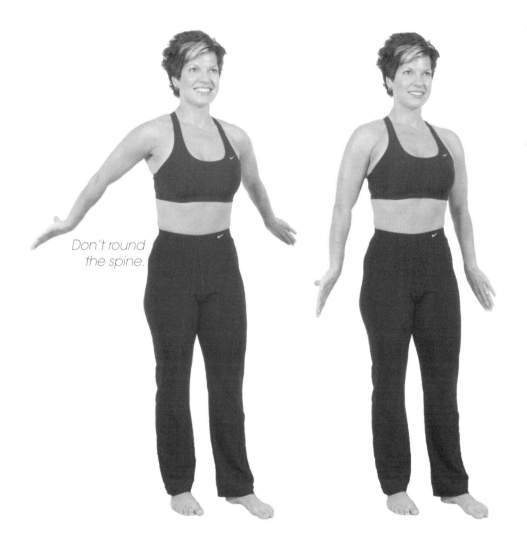

Don't round the spine.

Static Elbow Bend and Push

Triceps

Stand or sit tall. Lift one arm above the head. Bend the elbow and place the hand between the shoulder blades. Use the other hand to gently push the elbow back.

Hold the stretch for 10 to 30 seconds.

Repeat on the other arm.

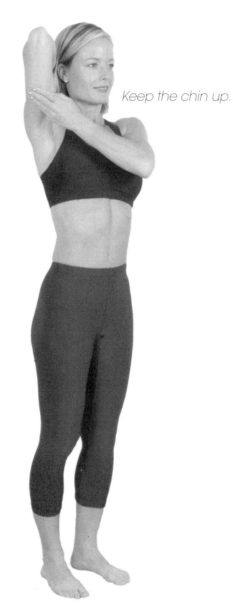

Keep the chin up.

ASSISTED STRETCH

Static Elbow Bend

Triceps

Stand or sit tall. Lift one arm above the head. Bend the elbow and place the hand between the shoulder blades as far down as comfortably possible.

Hold the stretch for 10 to 30 seconds.

Repeat on the other arm.

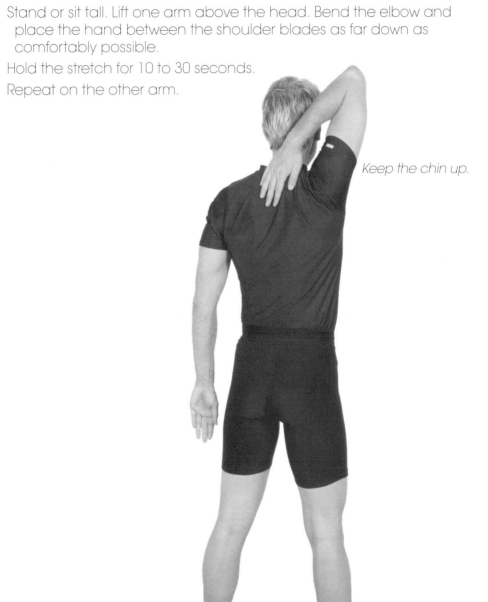

Keep the chin up.

Static Kneeling Elbow Push

Triceps

Kneel in front of a chair or platform. Place both hands on the back of the shoulder. Anchor the elbows on the chair or platform. Lean forward at the hip and bring the chest toward the floor.

Hold the stretch for 10 to 30 seconds.

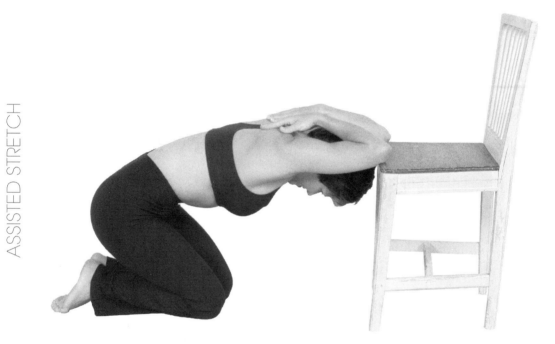

ASSISTED STRETCH

HANDS

In this day and age so many of us spend time using our forearms, wrists, and fingers to do tedious, repetitive tasks, such as typing on a keyboard, gripping a steering wheel, or using a cell phone. These stretches increase mobility in these areas and reverse the mechanical stress associated with hand and forearm overuse injuries.

Static Flex and Extend (wrists)

Wrists

Stand or sit with one hand in front of the body at shoulder height, palm facing down. Use the other hand to pull on the back of the hand, bringing the palm down toward the body. Return to setup position. Pull the hand up toward the body, bringing the back of the hand up.

Hold each stretch for 10 to 30 seconds.

Repeat on the other hand.

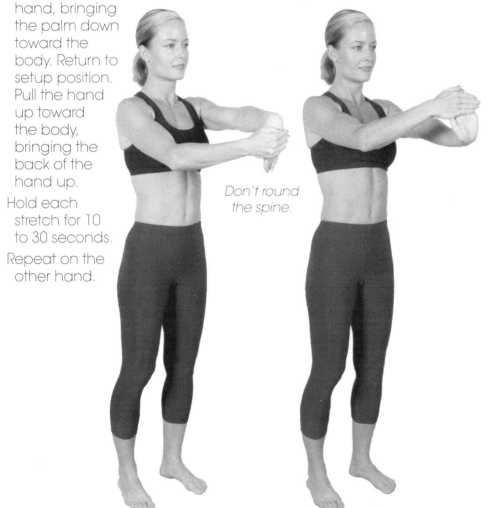

Don't round the spine.

Static Kneeling Flex and Extend (wrists)

Wrists

Kneel on the floor, lean forward, and place the palms of the hands on the floor with fingers pointing away from the body. Then turn the hands over with palms facing up; lean forward.

Hold each stretch for 10 to 30 seconds.

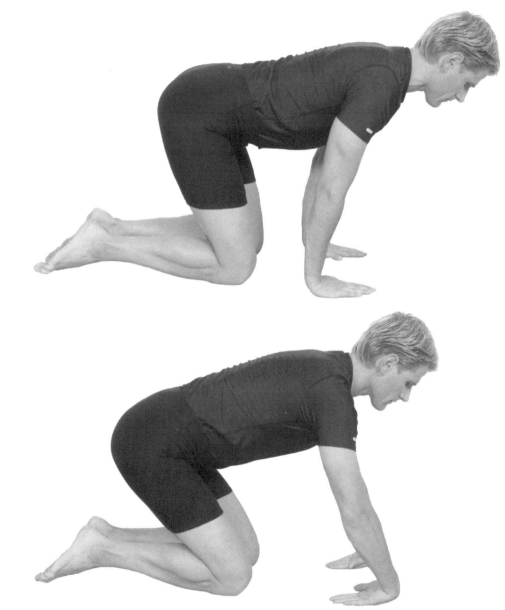

Dynamic Flex and Extend

Wrists

Stand or sit with arms held out in front at shoulder height and palms facing each other.

Start: Flex the wrists, turning the palms toward the body.

Finish: Extend the wrists, turning the palms away from the body.

Repeat as a continuous, controlled, fluid sequence 10 to 12 times.

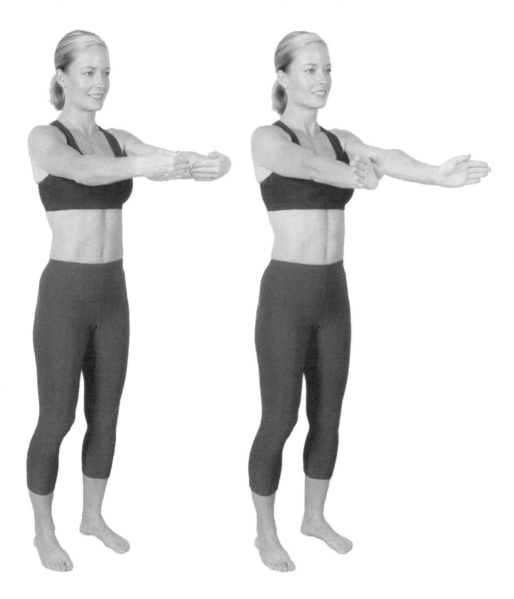

Dynamic Wrist Rolls

Wrists

Stand or sit with arms held out in front at shoulder height and palms facing down.

Start: Roll the hands in a clockwise, circular motion.

Finish: Roll the hands in a counterclockwise, circular motion.

Repeat as a continuous, controlled, fluid sequence 10 to 12 times.

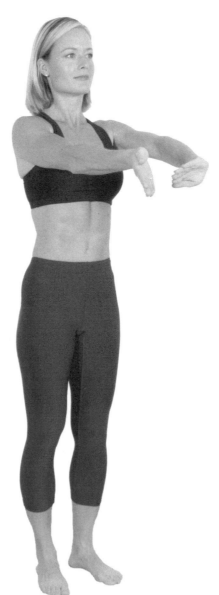

UNASSISTED STRETCH

Static Flex and Extend (fingers)

Fingers

Use one hand to push down and then pull back on the fingers of the other hand.

Hold the stretch for 10 to 30 seconds in both positions.

Repeat on the other hand.

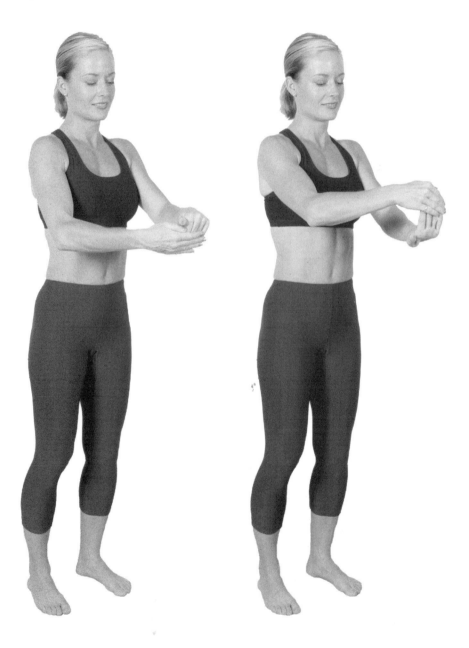

Static Kneeling Flex and Extend (fingers)

Fingers

Kneel on the floor; place the hands on the floor with the palms down. Push the hands toward the floor, keeping the fingers on the floor. Then place the back of the fingers on the floor and push the hands toward the floor.

Hold each stretch for 10 to 30 seconds.

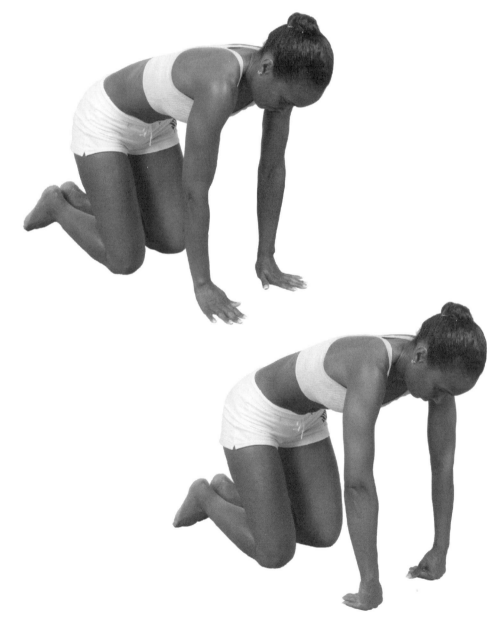

Dynamic Piano Fingers

Fingers

Stand or sit with arms held out in front of the body.

Wiggle the fingers in all directions as if playing the piano.

Repeat as a continuous, controlled, fluid sequence 10 to 12 times.

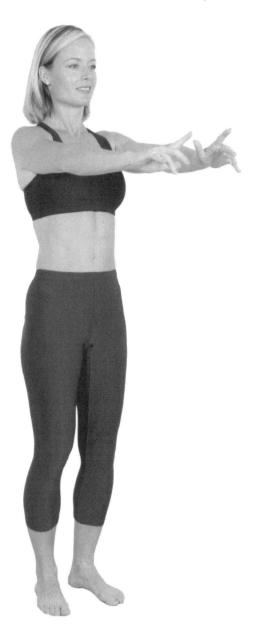

Dynamic Web Hands

Fingers

Stand or sit with arms held out in front of the body, palms facing away.

Start: Spread the fingers as far apart as comfortably possible.

Finish: Release the stretch by bringing the fingers together.

Repeat as a continuous, controlled, fluid sequence 10 to 12 times.

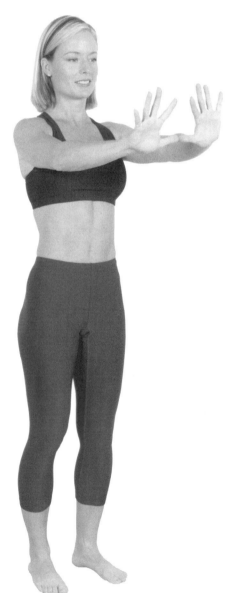

CHAPTER 3

Chest, Back, and Abdominals

In this chapter we'll focus on the muscles in the torso that work together to protect the spine, establish your posture, and develop your core. Muscle imbalance in your torso can lead to poor posture and a host of back problems; these muscles need to be strengthened and stretched frequently with the three-step system in mind.

CHEST

For most people, the muscles of the chest are tighter than the muscles in the back. This is because we spend most of the day working at our desks, driving our cars, carrying things, or reaching forward to pick things up. By performing stretches for the chest (especially dynamic, unassisted stretches), you can create a better balance between chest flexibility and back strength.

Static Kneeling Bow

Pectoralis

Kneeling on the floor, extend the arms directly out in front of the body while pushing the chest down toward the floor.

Hold the stretch for 10 to 30 seconds.

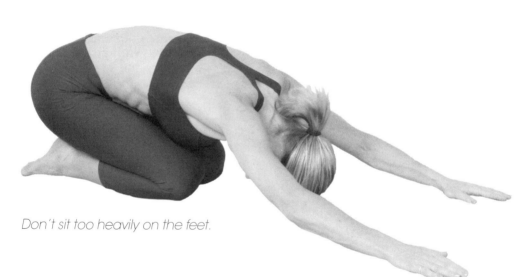

Don't sit too heavily on the feet.

Static Reach-Back and Turn

Pectoralis

Stand and raise the arm out to the side at shoulder height. Hold onto a stationary object, such as a door or cabinet. Slowly rotate the upper body away from the hand.

Hold the stretch for 10 to 30 seconds.

Repeat on the other arm.

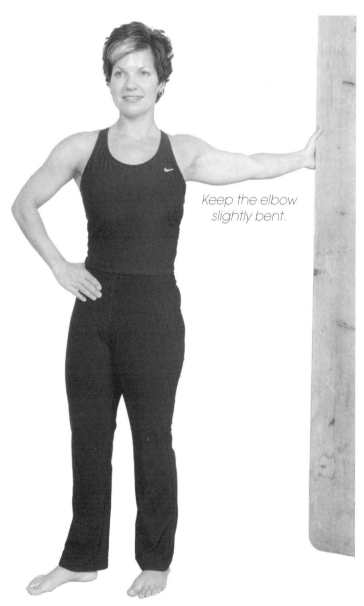

Keep the elbow slightly bent.

Static Chest Expansion

Pectoralis

Hold elbows at shoulder height with the fingers near the ears. Squeeze the shoulder blades together and pull the elbows back.

Hold the stretch for 10 to 30 seconds.

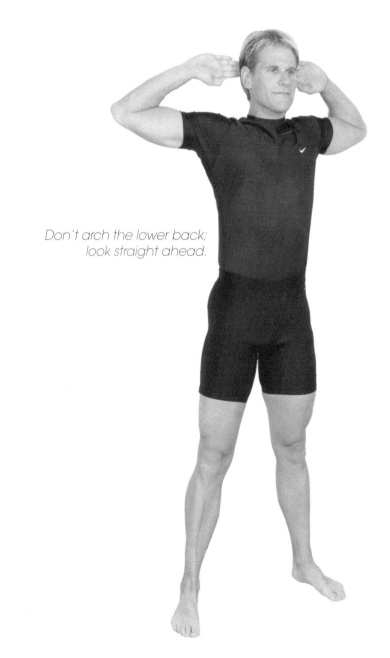

Don't arch the lower back; look straight ahead.

Dynamic Chest Expansion

Pectoralis

Hold elbows at shoulder height with the fingers near the ears.

Start: Squeeze the shoulder blades together and pull the elbows back.

Finish: Release the stretch by bringing the elbows in front of the ears.

Don't arch the lower back; continue looking straight ahead throughout the stretch.

Repeat as a continuous, controlled, fluid sequence 10 to 12 times.

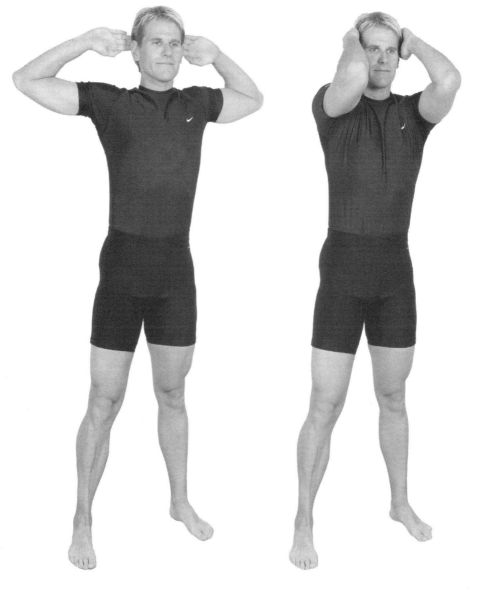

Dynamic Reach-Back and Turn

Pectoralis

Stand and raise one arm out to the side at shoulder height. Hold onto a stationary object, such as a door or cabinet.

Start: Slowly turn the upper body away from the hand, squeezing the shoulder blades together.

Finish: Release the stretch by bringing the upper body back to the setup position.

Repeat as a continuous, controlled, fluid sequence 10 to 12 times.

Repeat on the other arm.

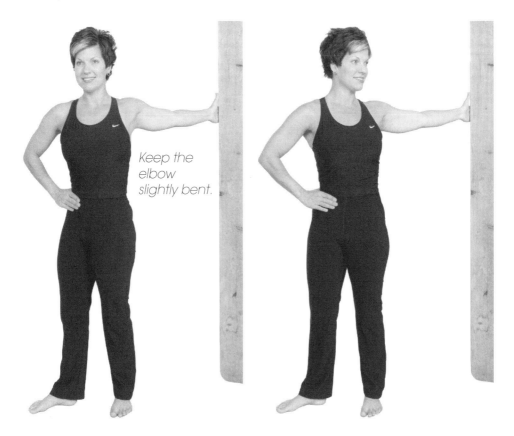

Keep the elbow slightly bent.

BACK

Back injuries are the second most comon medical complaint in the United States; headaches are the first. Although there's no one reason for back pain or injury, tightness and reduced mobility in the back are significant contributing factors. These stretches are designed to improve mobility in the back muscles and reduce tension in this very important area of the body.

Static Upper Scoop

Rhomboids (middle back)

Extend the legs straight in front with the knees slightly bent. Lean forward, reach for the back of the thighs, and round the upper back.

Hold the stretch for 10 to 30 seconds.

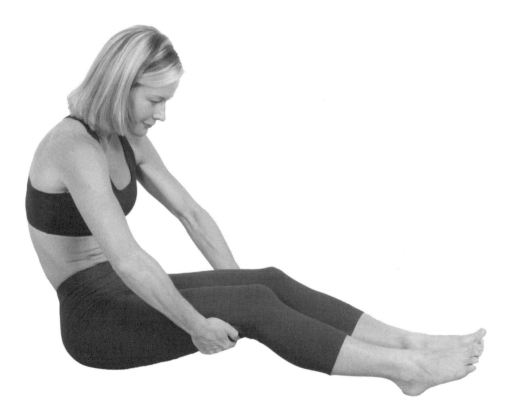

Dynamic Clasp and Round

Rhomboids (middle back)

Stand with the feet shoulder-width apart.

Start: Round the shoulders and reach forward with elbows bent. Clasp the hands together. Drop the chin toward the chest. Squeeze the chest to stretch the middle back.

Finish: Release the stretch by unlocking the hands; bring the arms out to the sides.

Repeat as a continuous, controlled, fluid sequence 10 to 12 times.

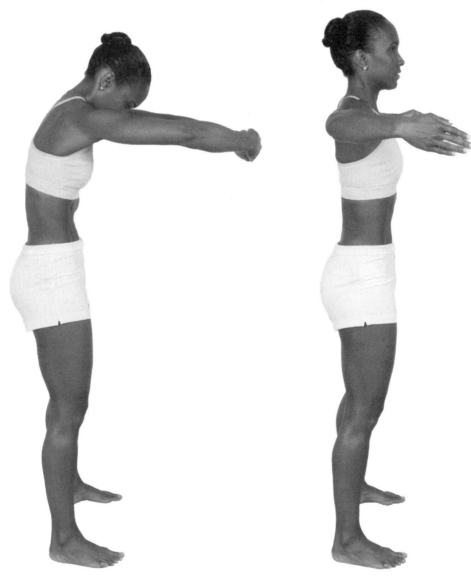

Static Seated Forward Bend

Trunk extensors (lower back)

Sit on the floor with the knees bent and legs wide. Drop the chest between the legs toward the floor.

Hold the stretch for 10 to 30 seconds.

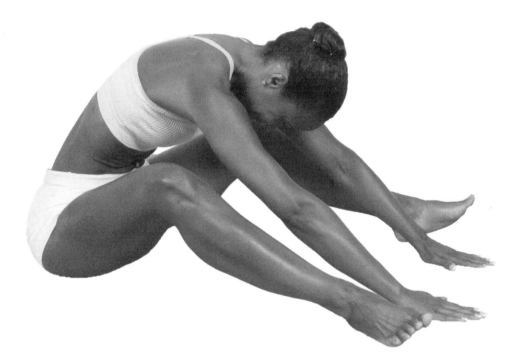

Static Lower Scoop

Trunk extensors (lower back)

Sit on the floor; extend the legs out in front with the knees slightly bent. Lean forward, hold the back of the thighs, and contract the abs to stretch the lower back.

Hold the stretch for 10 to 30 seconds.

UNASSISTED STRETCH

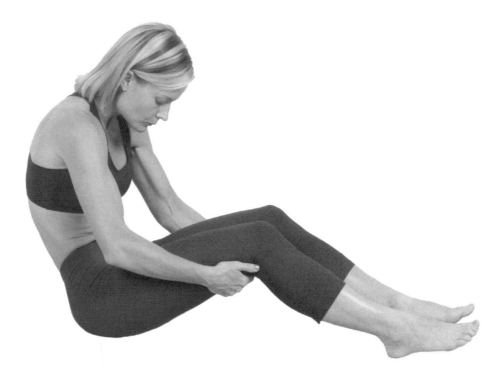

Dynamic Pelvic Tilt

Trunk extensors (lower back)

Stand with the feet shoulder-width apart.

Start: Contract the abs; tuck the tailbone underneath the spine.

Finish: Release the stretch by contracting the lower back; lift the tailbone out from underneath the spine.

Repeat as a continuous, controlled, fluid sequence 10 to 12 times.

Don't round or arch the middle or upper back.

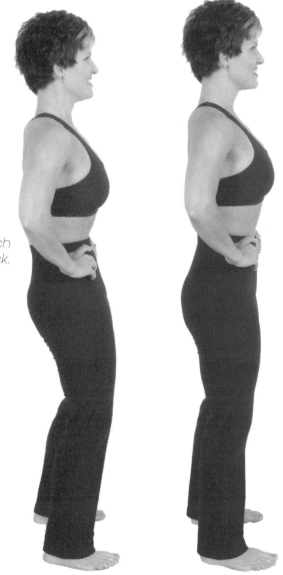

Dynamic Cat

Rhomboids, trunk extensors

Kneel on the floor on the hands and knees.

Start: Pull in the abdominals to round the spine; tuck the chin into the chest.

Finish: Release the stretch by returning to kneeling in the all-fours position.

Repeat as a continuous, controlled, fluid sequence 10 to 12 times.

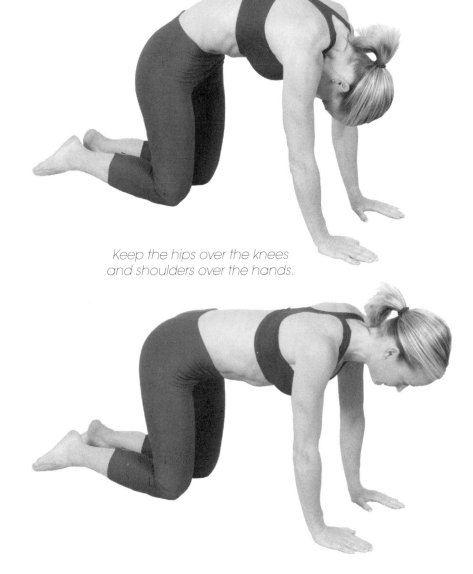

Keep the hips over the knees and shoulders over the hands.

Static Side Reach

Latissimus dorsi (side back), lateral trunk flexors (side lower back)

Stand with feet apart and knees slightly bent. Reach with one hand above the head and lean over to the opposite side.

Hold the stretch for 10 to 30 seconds.

Repeat on the other side.

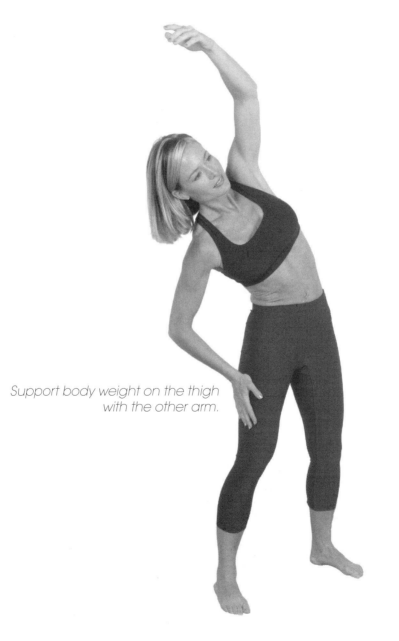

Support body weight on the thigh with the other arm.

Static Wall Reach

Latissimus dorsi (side back), lateral trunk flexors (side lower back)

Stand with the feet apart. With one side of the body facing the wall, place both hands on the wall by leaning to the side.

Hold the stretch for 10 to 30 seconds.

Repeat on the other side.

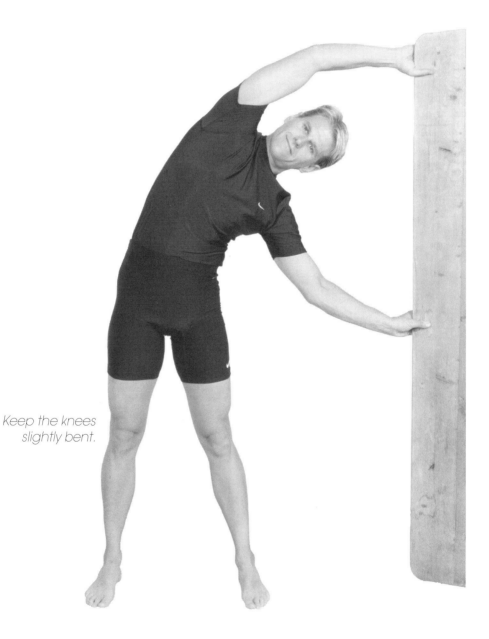

Keep the knees slightly bent.

ASSISTED STRETCH

Dynamic Side Reach

Latissimus dorsi (side back), lateral trunk flexors (side lower back)

Stand with feet apart and knees slightly bent.

Start: Reach with one hand above the head; lean over to the opposite side.

Finish: Reach with the other hand to the opposite side.

Use the other arm to support the body weight on the thigh, if necessary.

Repeat as a continuous, controlled, fluid sequence 10 to 12 times.

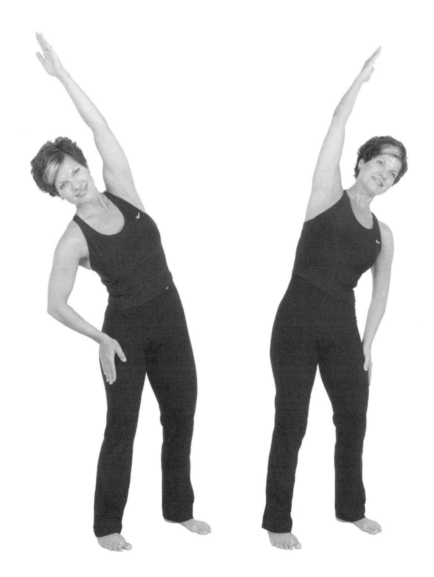

Static Seated Twist

Thoracic-lumbar rotators

Sitting on the floor, extend the legs straight out in front with the knees slightly bent. Place one hand on the floor behind the body and the other across the thigh. Twist the upper body to one side.

Hold the stretch for 10 to 30 seconds.

Repeat on the other side.

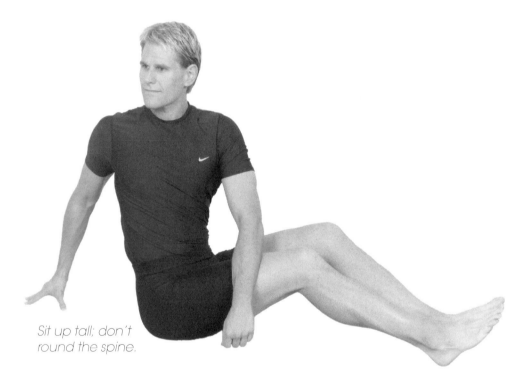

Sit up tall; don't round the spine.

Dynamic Twist

Thoracic-lumbar rotators

Stand with feet shoulder-width apart. Bend the elbows; hold the arms out to the sides.

Start: Twist the upper body to one side.

Finish: Twist the upper body to the opposite side.

Repeat as a continuous, controlled, fluid sequence 10 to 12 times.

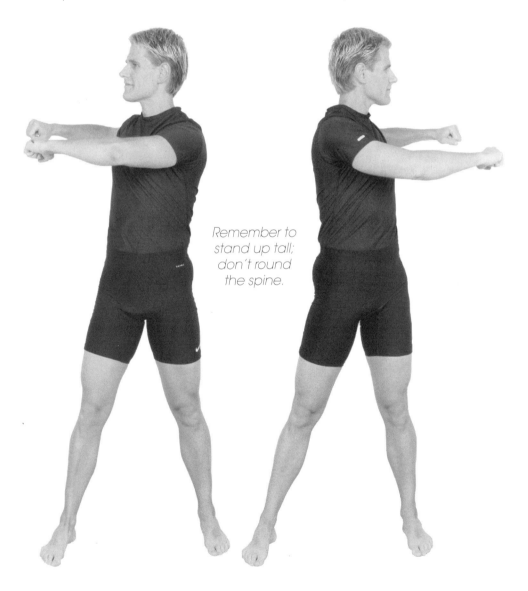

Remember to stand up tall; don't round the spine.

ABDOMINALS

Along with the muscles of the lower back, the abdominal muscles help to hold us upright throughout the day. They are essential for supporting and protecting the spine. Performing abdominal stretches helps keep your abdominal muscles flexible and strong, which aids everyday movement and function.

Static Cobra

Abdominals

Lie on the floor chest down with the hands near the shoulders. Lift the chest and ribs off the floor as far as comfortably possible by pushing with the hands.

Don't extend beyond the point that's comfortable for the lower back.

Hold the stretch for 10 to 30 seconds.

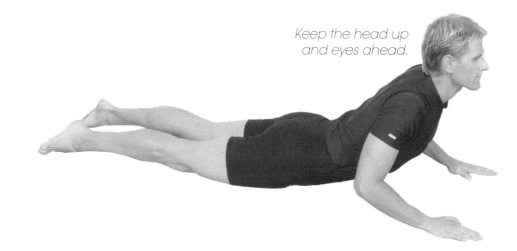

Keep the head up and eyes ahead.

Static Roll on Ball

Abdominals

Place the middle back on the center of a stability ball with the feet out in front and the hands interlaced behind the head. Lower the tailbone, upper back, and head around the ball.

Hold the stretch for 10 to 30 seconds.

Don't extend beyond the point that's comfortable for the lower back.

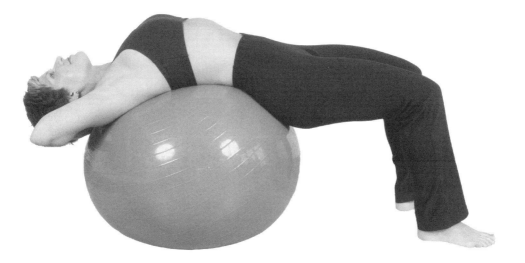

Static Lying Arch

Abdominals

Lie on the floor face up with the arms extended above the head. Reach as far away from the body as comfortably possible while gently arching the lower back and lifting the ribs and chest toward the ceiling.

Hold the stretch for 10 to 30 seconds.

Don't extend beyond the point that's comfortable for the lower back.

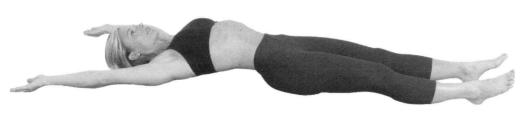

Dynamic Cobra

Abdominals

Lie on the floor face down with the hands in front of the body.

Start: Lift the chest and ribs off the floor by contracting the back muscles.

Finish: Release the stretch by returning to the setup position.

Repeat as a continuous, controlled, fluid sequence 10 to 12 times.

Don't extend beyond the point that's comfortable for the lower back.

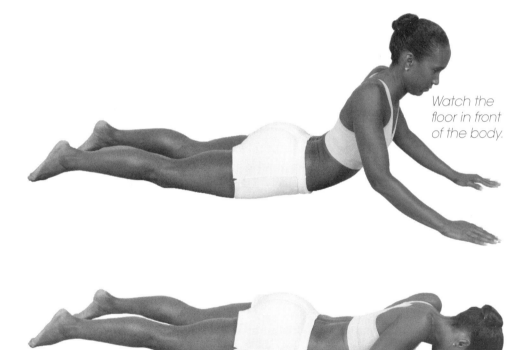

Watch the floor in front of the body.

Dynamic Arch

Abdominals

Stand tall with the palms of the hands around the sides of the lower back.

Start: Lift the chest and ribs toward the ceiling by contracting the back muscles and extending the spine.

Finish: Release the stretch by returning to the setup position.

Repeat as a continuous, controlled, fluid sequence 10 to 12 times.

Don't extend beyond the point that's comfortable for the lower back.

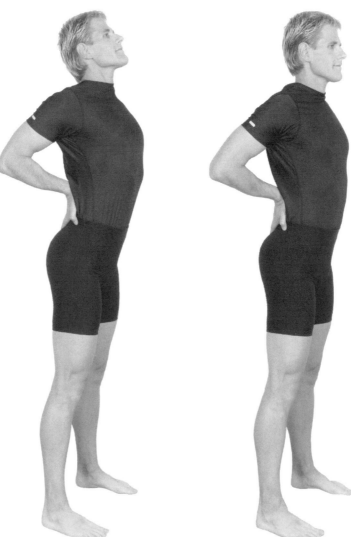

CHAPTER 4

Buttocks, Hips, Quadriceps, and Hamstrings

In this chapter we'll focus on the large muscles that surround the pelvis and upper leg. These muscles are among the strongest and most powerful in the body. They also tend to be among the tightest. Poor mobility in these muscles can lead to problems that travel up the body into the back or down the lower body into the knees. The stretches in this chapter supply relief and strength to this very important region of the body.

BUTTOCKS AND HIPS

The buttocks and hips comprise a great number of muscles that engage every time you sit down, stand up, or climb the stairs. These muscles also work to stabilize the pelvis for many other activities, such as bending over or leaning sideways. Stretching these muscles frequently helps counteract all the stress these activities create for this area of the body.

Static Lying Figure 4

Gluteals, piriformis

Lie on the floor with the legs bent. Place one foot across the thigh of the opposite leg in the figure 4 position. Reach for the leg on the floor and pull it toward the chest.

Hold the stretch for 10 to 30 seconds.

Repeat on the other leg.

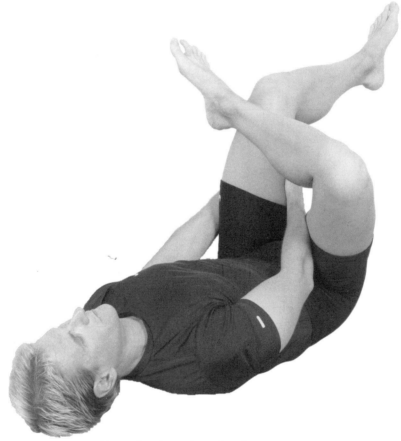

Keep the head on the floor.

Static Seated Figure 4

Gluteals, piriformis

Sitting on the floor, extend one leg straight out in front; put the foot of the other leg across the thigh in the figure 4 position. Move the chest toward the legs, pivoting at the hip.

Hold the stretch for 10 to 30 seconds.

Repeat on the other leg.

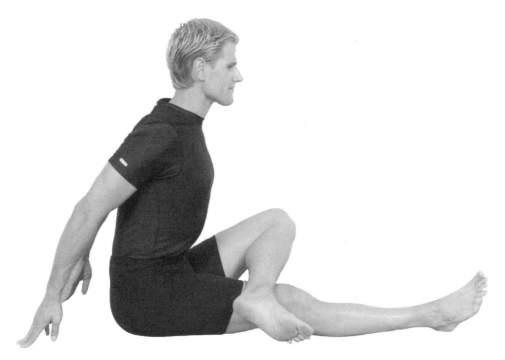

Use the arms to support the back.

Static Seated Figure 4 (on chair)

Gluteals, piriformis

Sit in a chair with one foot across the thigh of the opposite leg in the figure 4 position. Move the chest toward the legs, pivoting at the hip. Use the arms to support the back, if necessary.

Hold the stretch for 10 to 30 seconds.

Repeat on the other leg.

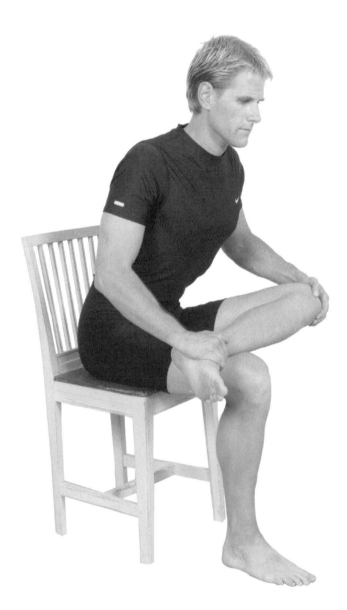

Static Dancer

Gluteals, piriformis

Lie face down. Raise the upper body off the floor, resting on elbows. Bend one knee and bring it underneath the opposite leg. Lower the upper body toward the floor.

Hold the stretch for 10 to 30 seconds.

Repeat on the other leg.

Relax the head and neck.

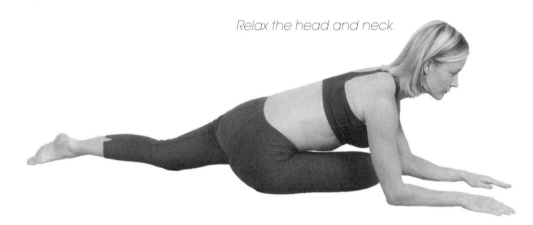

Static Figure 4

Gluteals, piriformis

Stand with feet slightly apart. Place one foot across the thigh of the opposite leg in the figure 4 position. Squat down.

Hold onto a chair for balance, if necessary.

Hold the stretch for 10 to 30 seconds.

Repeat on the other leg.

Keep the head up;
don't round the spine.

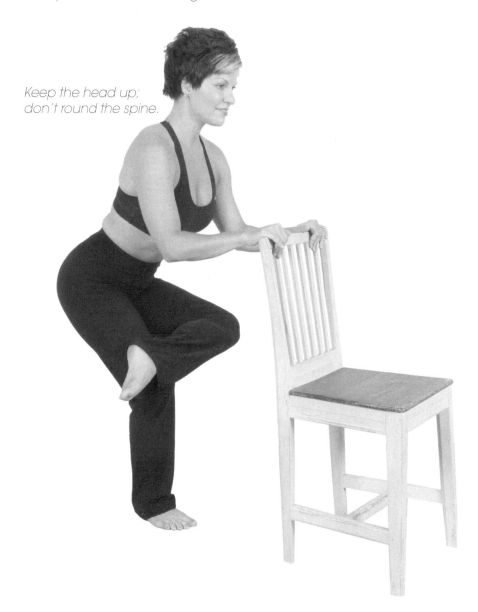

Static Hip Push

Gluteals, piriformis

Stand with feet together; hold onto a chair. Bend forward slightly at the waist. Bend one leg and straighten the other, pushing the straight leg hip outward.

Hold the stretch for 10 to 30 seconds.

Repeat on the other leg.

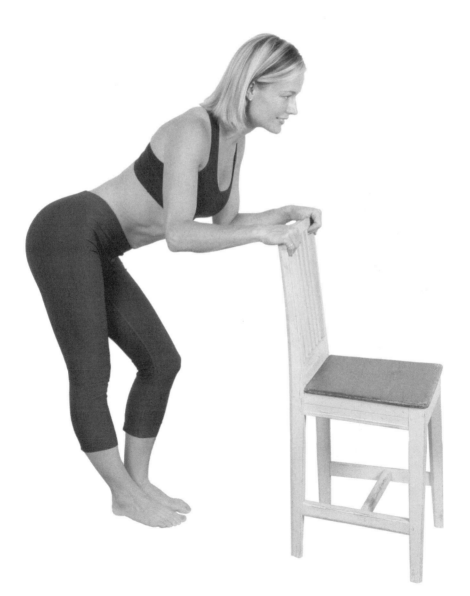

Dynamic Knee Hug

Gluteals

Stand with feet together. Bring one knee forward and up toward the chest.

Start: Place the hands around the shin and pull the knee into the chest.

Finish: Release the stretch by putting the foot on the floor. Repeat with the opposite leg.

Repeat as a continuous, controlled, fluid sequence 10 to 12 times, alternating legs.

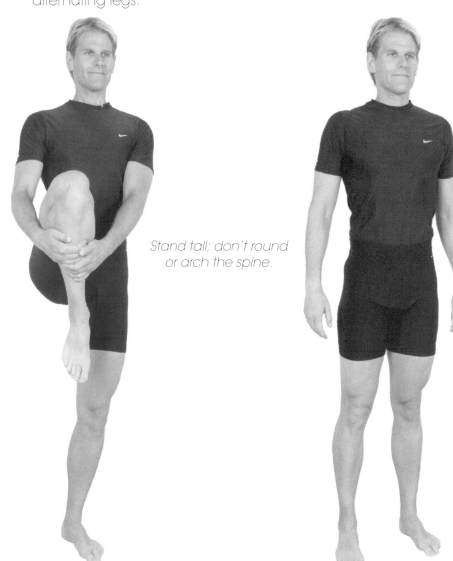

Stand tall; don't round or arch the spine.

Dynamic Lying Figure 4 Circles

Gluteals, piriformis

Lie on the floor on the back with the knees bent. Place one foot across the thigh of the opposite leg in the figure 4 position. Lift the other foot off the floor and rotate the leg in a circular motion. Repeat as a continuous, controlled, fluid sequence 10 to 12 times.

Repeat on the other leg.

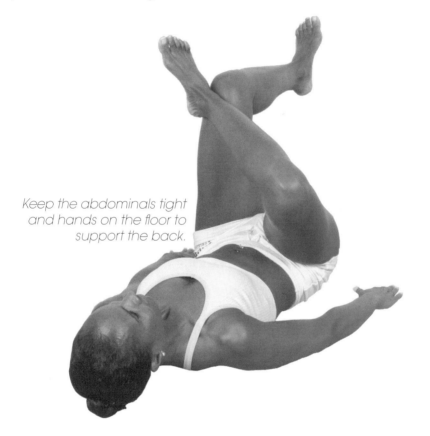

Keep the abdominals tight and hands on the floor to support the back.

Dynamic Hip Push

Gluteals, piriformis

Standing with the feet together, bend the elbows and hold onto a chair with the hands. Bend forward slightly at the waist.

Start: Bend one leg and straighten the other, pushing the straight leg hip outward.

Finish: Switch to the other side.

Repeat as a continuous, controlled, fluid sequence 10 to 12 times.

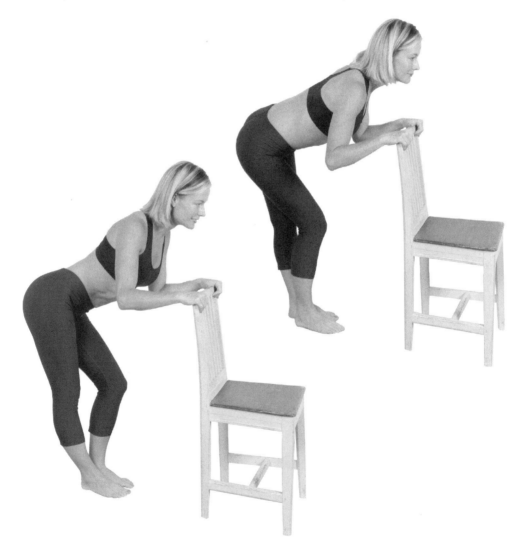

Static Lying Crossover

Internal hip rotators

Lie on the back with the knees bent, soles of the feet on the floor, and knees touching. Lift one leg slightly, and drop the other knee inward toward the floor.

Hold the stretch for 10 to 30 seconds.

Repeat on the other leg.

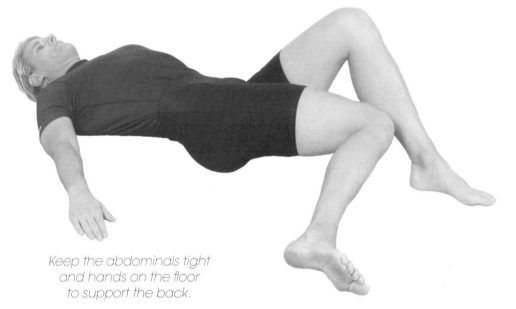

Keep the abdominals tight and hands on the floor to support the back.

Dynamic Lying Crossover

Internal hip rotators

Lie on the back with the knees bent, soles of the feet on the floor, and knees touching.

Start: Lift one leg slightly, and drop the other knee inward toward the floor.

Finish: Release the stretch by switching to the opposite side.

Repeat as a continuous, controlled, fluid sequence 10 to 12 times.

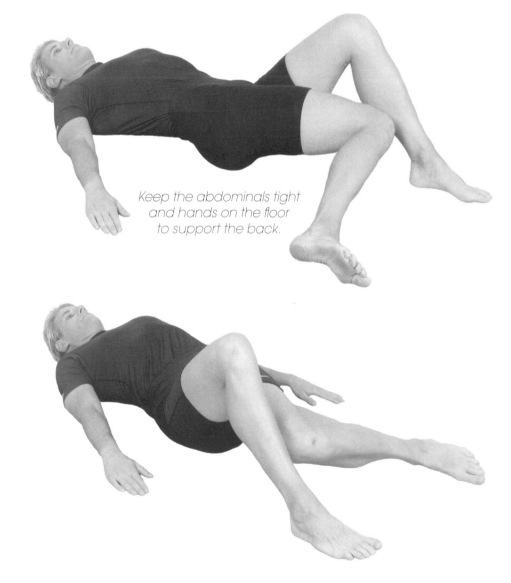

Keep the abdominals tight and hands on the floor to support the back.

Static Lunge

Hip flexors

Stand tall with legs in a lunge position. Lower the back knee toward the floor and tilt the hips toward the ceiling.

Hold the stretch for 10 to 30 seconds.

Repeat on the other leg.

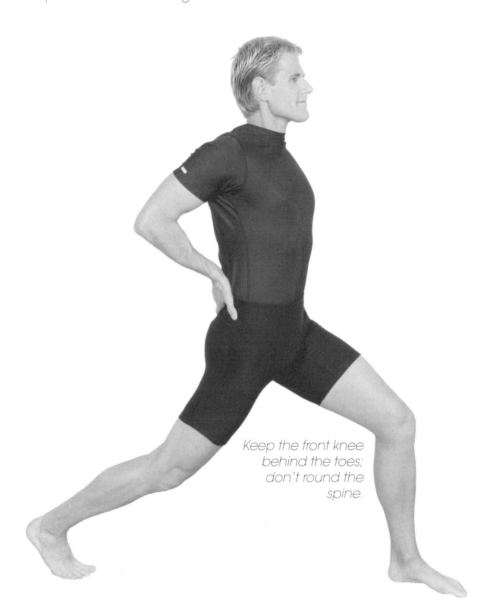

Keep the front knee behind the toes; don't round the spine.

Static Kneeling Runner's Lunge

Hip flexors

Kneel on one leg. Step out with the front foot and gently press the hips forward.

Place the hands on the front thigh for support, if necessary.

Keep body weight distributed between both legs.

Hold the stretch for 10 to 30 seconds.

Repeat on the other leg.

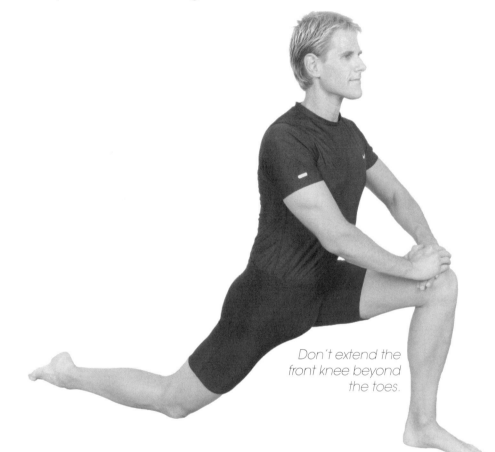

Don't extend the front knee beyond the toes.

Static Anchored Lunge

Hip flexors

Stand tall and place one foot behind you on a chair or bench. Bend the front leg and push the hips forward.

Hold the stretch for 10 to 30 seconds.

Repeat on the other leg.

Don't extend the front knee beyond the toes.

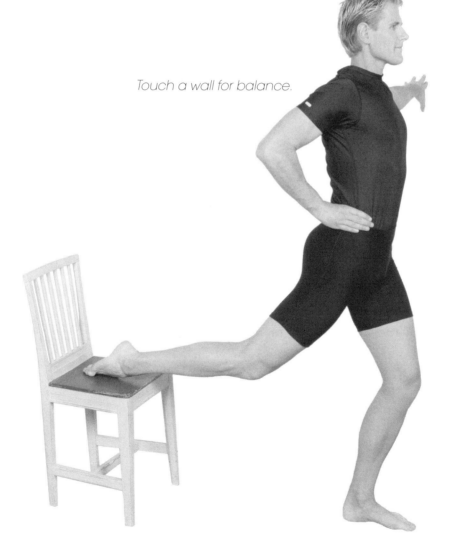

Touch a wall for balance.

Dynamic Lying Leg Lift

Hip flexors

Lie on the belly with the head turned to one side. Bend one knee until the sole of the foot faces the ceiling.

Start: Lift the front of the thigh off the floor as high as comfortably possible.

Finish: Release the stretch by lowering the thigh back to the floor.

Repeat as a continuous, controlled, fluid sequence 10 to 12 times.

Repeat on the other leg.

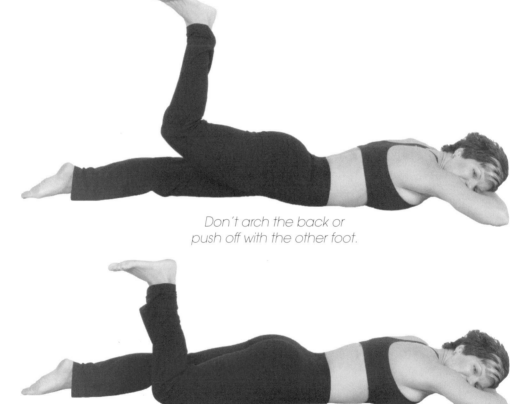

*Don't arch the back or
push off with the other foot.*

Dynamic Hip Extension

Hip flexors

Stand tall.

Start: Straighten one leg and extend it behind the body as far as comfortably possible.

Finish: Release the stretch by returning to the setup position.

Repeat as a continuous, controlled, fluid sequence 10 to 12 times. Repeat on the other leg.

Touch a wall or hold onto something for balance, if necessary.

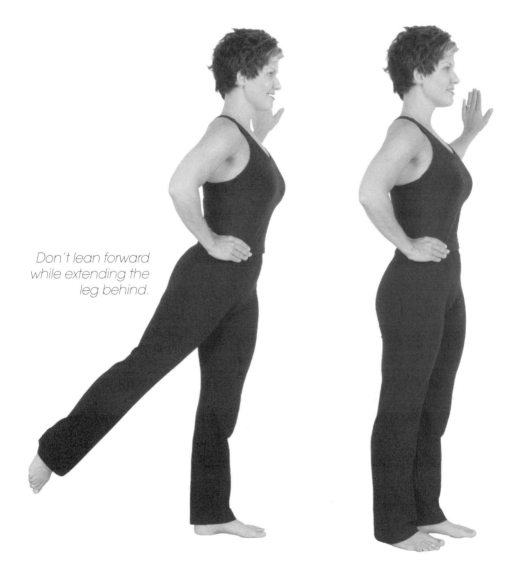

Don't lean forward while extending the leg behind.

INNER THIGH

The muscles of the inner thigh tend to be tight and weak for many people because of lack of use. The risk associated with tight or weak inner thigh muscles is minimal in typical daily activities but proves very important if you're involved in activities such as in-line skating or horseback riding. Strong and stretched inner thigh muscles help prevent falls and groin injuries.

Static Seated Butterfly

Adductors

Sit on the floor with the soles of the feet together. Place the forearms or elbows on the inner thighs; bring the chest slightly toward the legs. Pivot from the hips and push the thighs toward the floor.

Hold the stretch for 10 to 30 seconds.

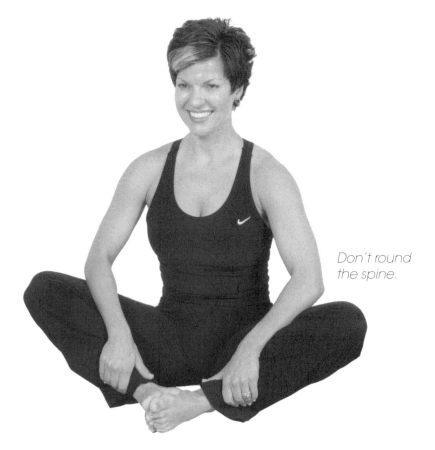

Don't round the spine.

ASSISTED STRETCH

Static Side Lunge

Adductors

Stand with feet wide apart. Bend one knee and lunge to the same side, keeping the other leg straight.

Don't round the spine.

Hold the stretch for 10 to 30 seconds.

Repeat on the other side.

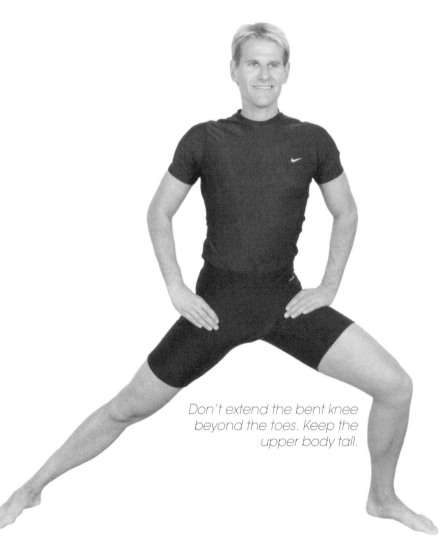

Don't extend the bent knee beyond the toes. Keep the upper body tall.

Static Sumo Squat

ASSISTED STRETCH

Adductors

Stand with feet wide apart, toes turned out at a diagonal from the body. Sit down into a low squat position. Lean forward and use the forearms to press against the inside of the thighs.

Hold the stretch for 10 to 30 seconds.

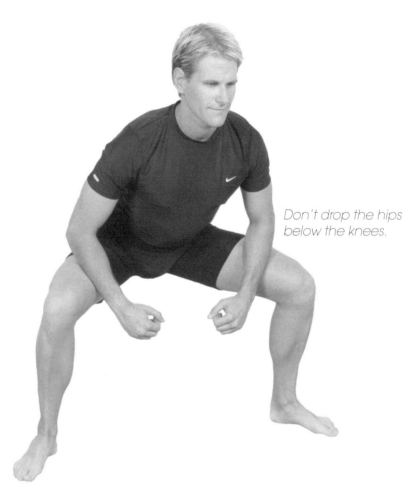

Don't drop the hips below the knees.

Static Lying Straddle

Adductors

Lie on the floor with the legs in the air and the knees slightly bent.
Slowly open the legs and lower them toward the floor.

Hold the stretch for 10 to 30 seconds.

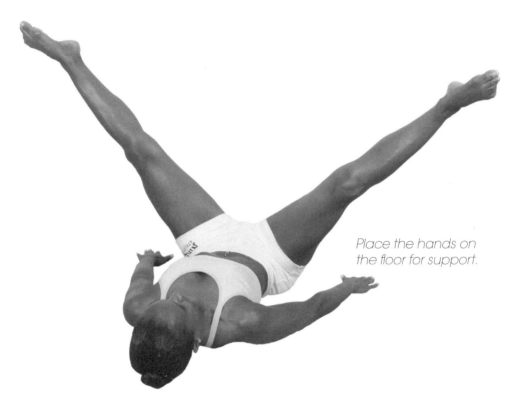

*Place the hands on
the floor for support.*

Static Seated Straddle

Adductors

Extend the legs straight out in front with knees very slightly bent. Open the legs as wide as comfortably possible.

Hold the stretch for 10 to 30 seconds.

Use the arms to support the back.

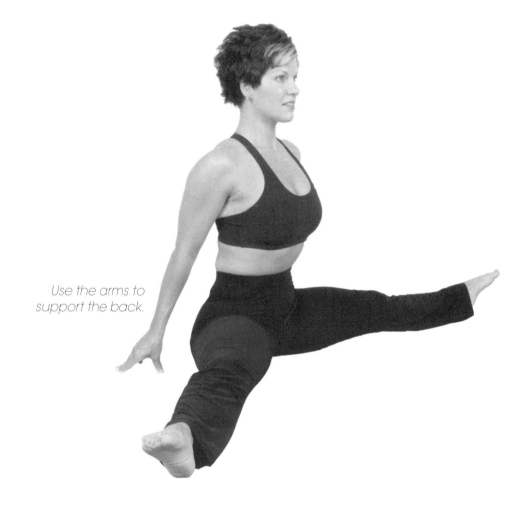

Static Frog Straddle

Adductors

Kneeling on the floor, keep the feet together and open the knees as wide as comfortably possible. Rest the upper body on the elbows.

Hold the stretch for 10 to 30 seconds.

Don't arch the back.

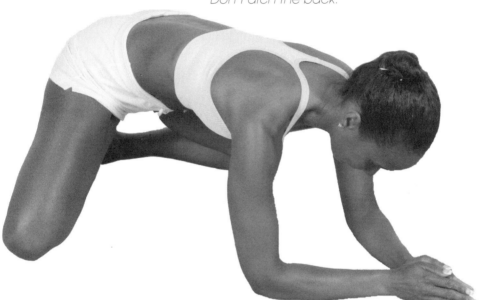

Dynamic Seated Butterfly

Adductors

Sit on the floor and bring the soles of the feet together.

Start: Pull the knees to the floor by contracting the outside of the thighs.

Finish: Release the legs to the setup position.

Repeat as a continuous, controlled, fluid sequence 10 to 12 times.

Use the arms to support the back, if necessary.

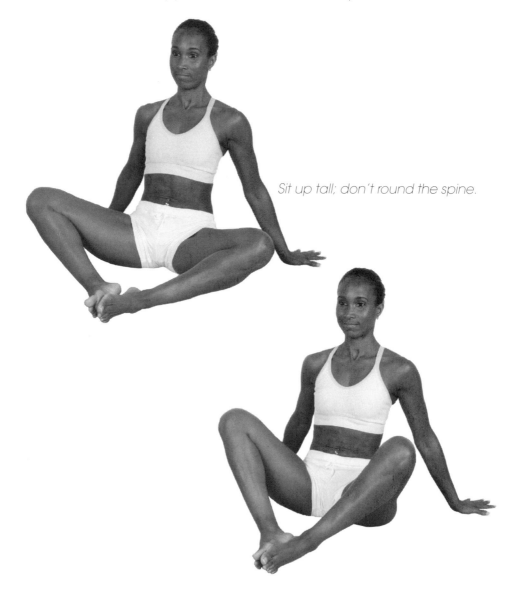

Sit up tall; don't round the spine.

Dynamic Side Lunge

Adductors

Stand with feet wide apart.

Start: Bend one knee and lunge to the same side. Contract the gluteals on the opposite side and keep that leg straight.

Finish: Switch sides.

Repeat as a continuous, controlled, fluid sequence 10 to 12 times.

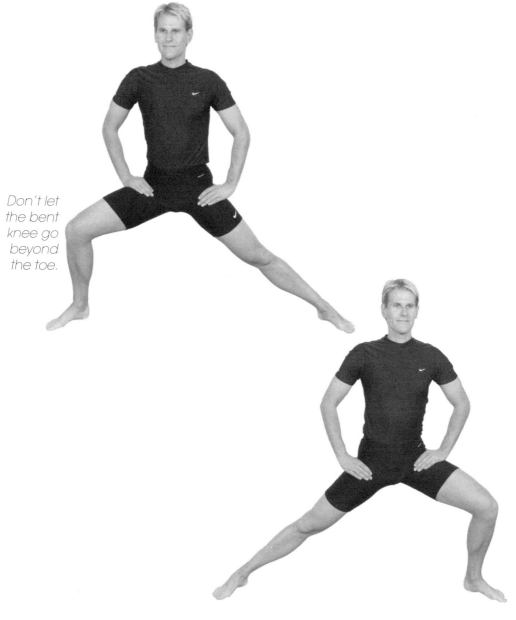

Don't let the bent knee go beyond the toe.

Dynamic Seated Straddle

Adductors

Extend the legs straight in front of you with the knees slightly bent. Open the legs as wide as possible.

Start: Contract the gluteals. Lean forward, pivoting at the hips.

Finish: Release the stretch by lifting the upper body to an upright position.

Repeat as a continuous, controlled, fluid sequence 10 to 12 times.

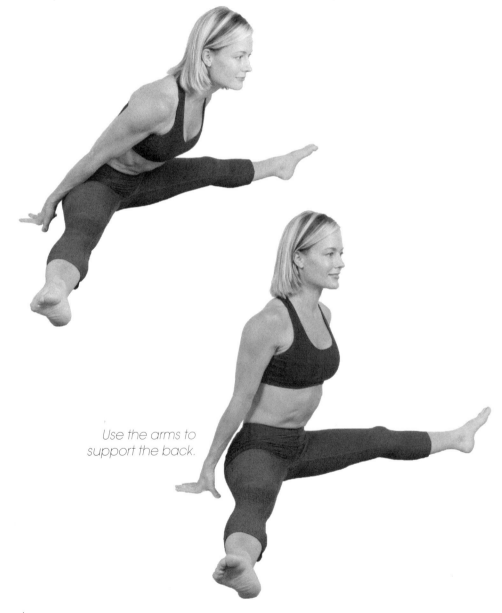

Use the arms to support the back.

Dynamic Side Leg Lift

Adductors

Standing with the feet together, touch the back of a chair with the palms of the hands.

Start: Raise one leg out to the side as high as comfortably possible.

Finish: Release the stretch by lowering the leg to the floor.

Repeat as a continuous, controlled, fluid sequence 10 to 12 times.

Repeat on the other leg.

Keep the upper body tall.

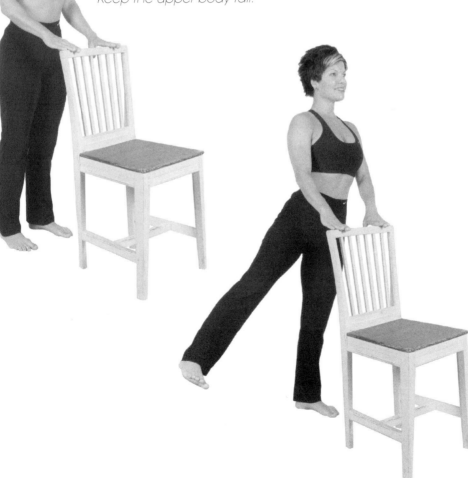

FRONT THIGH (QUADRICEPS)

The quadriceps is a large group of four very strong muscles that make up the front of the thigh. We use them in nearly every sport and when we stand, sit, or walk. Although the quads are not tight for most people, they are worked hard every day and are often fatigued. Stretching these muscles feels good and improves mobility around the knee joint.

Static Knee Bend

Quadriceps

Stand with feet together. Bend one knee and hold the ankle with the same-side hand; pull the heel toward the gluteals.

Hold the stretch for 10 to 30 seconds.

Repeat on the other leg.

Touch a wall or hold onto something for balance, if necessary.

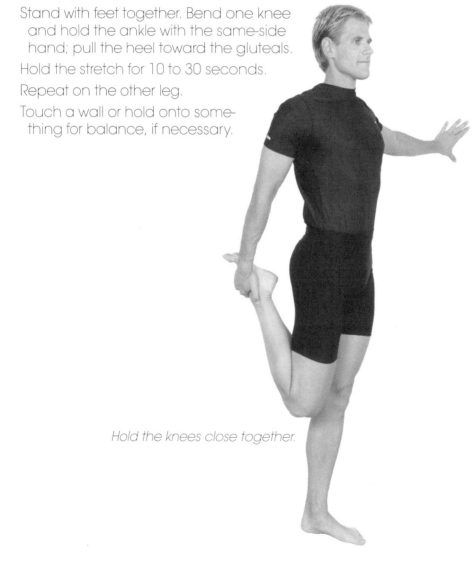

Hold the knees close together.

Static Side-Lying Knee Bend

Quadriceps

Lie on one side and rest the head on the lower arm. Bend the top knee and hold the ankle with the same-side hand; pull the heel toward the gluteals.

Hold the stretch for 10 to 30 seconds.

Repeat on the other leg.

Remember to hold the knees close together.

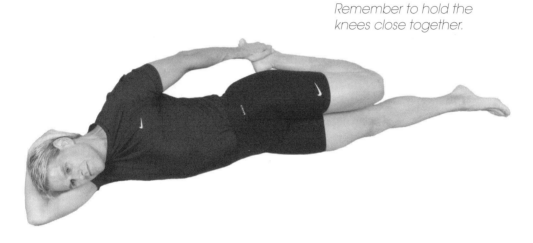

Static Anchored Knee Bend

Quadriceps

Stand with feet together, facing away from the back of a chair. Bend one knee and place the top of the foot on the back of the chair.

Hold the stretch for 10 to 30 seconds.

Repeat on the other leg.

Touch a wall or hold onto something for balance, if necessary.

Hold the knees close together.

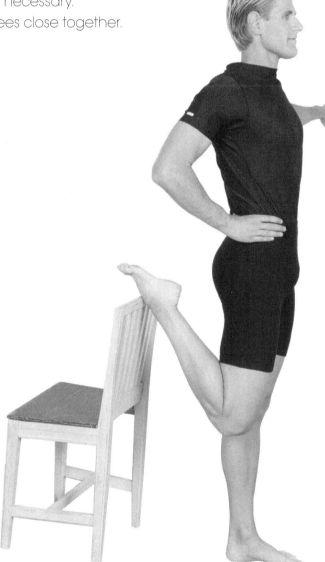

Dynamic Side-Lying Knee Bend

Quadriceps

Lie on one side and rest the head in the palm of the lower hand.

Start: Bend the top leg at the knee, bringing the heel toward the gluteals.

Finish: Release the stretch by returning the leg to the setup position.

Repeat as a continuous, controlled, fluid sequence 10 to 12 times.

Repeat on the other leg.

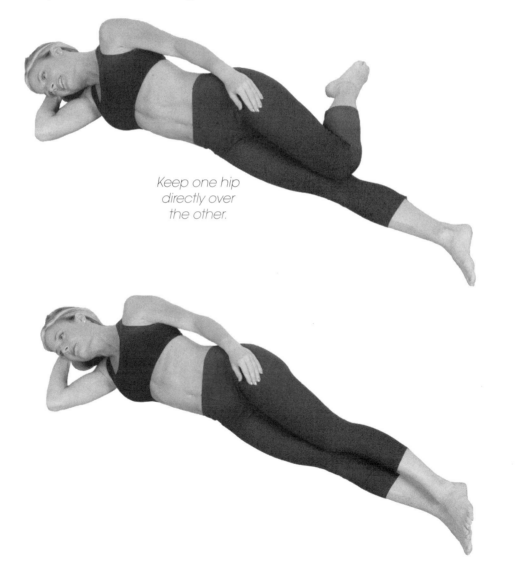

Keep one hip directly over the other.

Dynamic Lying Knee Bend

Quadriceps

Lie face down with legs extended and the head turned to one side resting on the tops of the hands.

Start: Bend the knee on one leg and move the heel toward the gluteals.

Finish: Release the stretch by returning the leg to the setup position.

Repeat as a continuous, controlled, fluid sequence 10 to 12 times.

Repeat on the other leg.

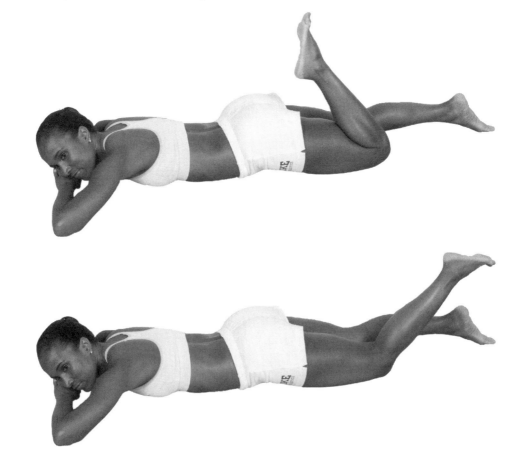

UNASSISTED STRETCH

Dynamic Knee Bend

Quadriceps

Stand with the feet together.

Start: Raise the heel of one foot toward the buttocks.

Finish: Release the stretch by returning the leg to the setup position.

Repeat as a continuous, controlled, fluid sequence 10 to 12 times.

Repeat on the other leg.

Hold onto a chair for balance, if necessary.

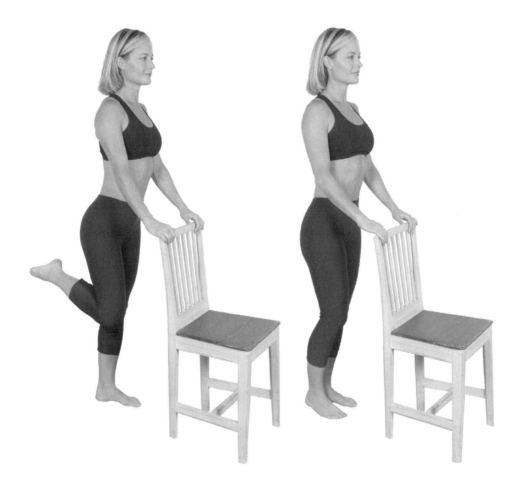

HAMSTRINGS

The hamstring muscles make up the back of the upper thigh. They work in partnership with the quadriceps to bend and straighten the knee and extend the hip. Many people have tight hamstrings from sitting so much during the day (the seated position shortens the hamstrings). Strong and flexible hamstrings improve mobility around the hip joint and make almost all activities easier and more comfortable.

Static Lying Scissor

Hamstrings

Lie on the floor face up with legs slightly bent. Lift one leg, keeping the knee straight. Place hands (or a strap) around the thigh and move the leg closer to the head.

Hold the stretch for 10 to 30 seconds.

Repeat on the other leg.

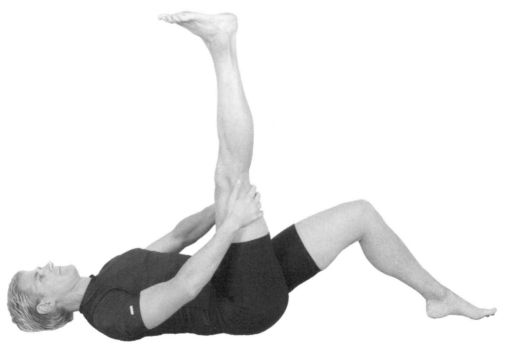

Don't round the spine.

ASSISTED STRETCH

Static One-Leg Hip Hinge

Hamstrings

Stand with one foot forward and one foot back. Straighten the front leg and bend the back knee. Lean forward, pivoting at the hips, and place the hands on the thigh of the bent knee.

Hold the stretch for 10 to 30 seconds.

Repeat on the other leg.

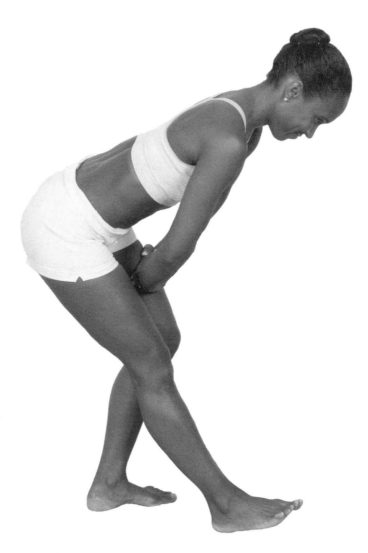

Static Two-Leg Hip Hinge

Hamstrings

Stand with feet together facing a wall or chair. Lean forward, pivoting at the hips. Keep the knees straight but not locked. Use the wall or chair to hold you in place.

Hold the stretch for 10 to 30 seconds.

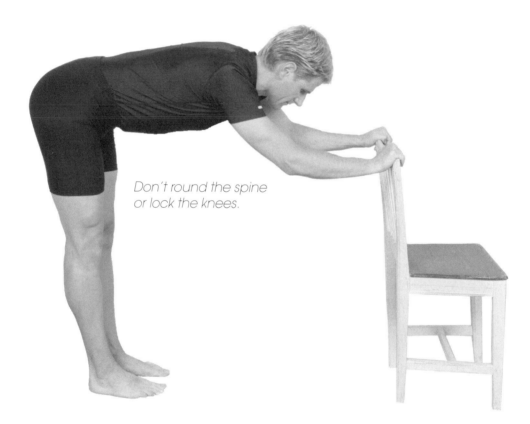

Don't round the spine or lock the knees.

Static Leg Up

Hamstrings

Stand with feet together facing the back of a chair. Raise one leg and rest it on top of the back of the chair. Stand tall and straighten the knee.

Hold the stretch for 10 to 30 seconds.

Repeat on the other leg.

Touch a wall or hold onto something for balance, if necessary.

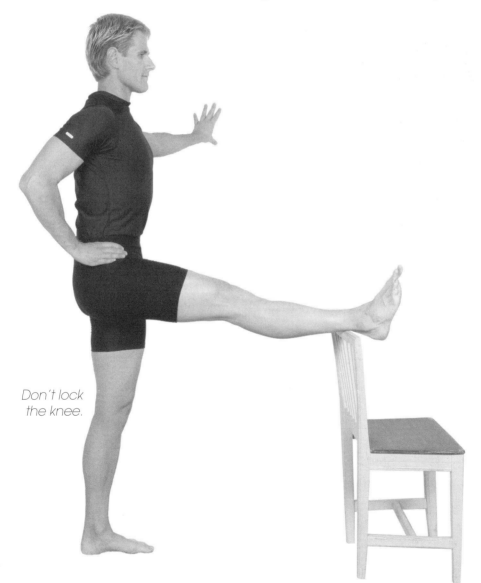

Don't lock the knee.

Dynamic Knee Kick

Hamstrings

Stand tall and lift one leg up to hip height, keeping the knee bent.

Start: Straighten the knee.

Finish: Release the stretch by bending the knee.

Repeat as a continuous, controlled, fluid sequence 10 to 12 times.

Repeat on the other leg.

Touch a wall or hold onto something for balance, if necessary.

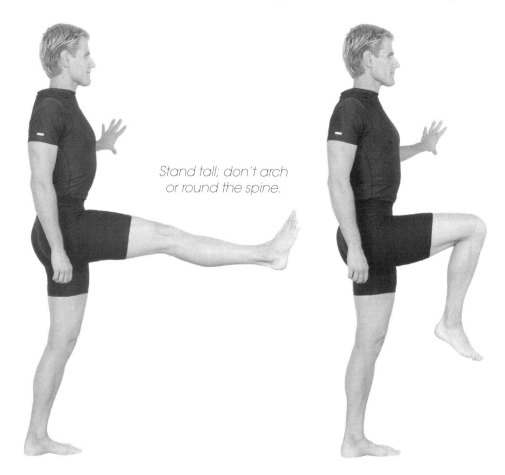

Stand tall; don't arch or round the spine.

Dynamic Lying Scissor

Hamstrings

Lie on the floor face up with legs slightly bent.

Start: Lift one leg as close to the body as comfortably possible, keeping the knee straight.

Finish: Release the stretch by slowly lowering the leg to the floor.

Repeat as a continuous, controlled, fluid sequence 10 to 12 times.

Repeat on the other leg.

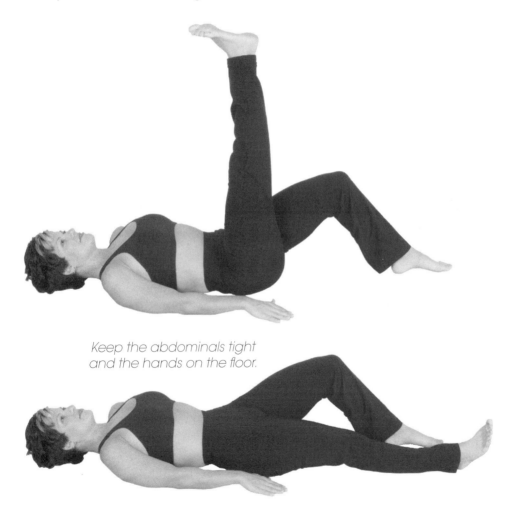

Keep the abdominals tight and the hands on the floor.

Dynamic Lying Knee Kick

Hamstrings

Lie on the floor face up holding one leg up with the knee bent.

Start: Straighten the knee as much as comfortably possible.

Finish: Release the stretch by bending the knee back to the setup position.

Repeat as a continuous, controlled, fluid sequence 10 to 12 times.

Repeat on the other leg.

UNASSISTED STRETCH

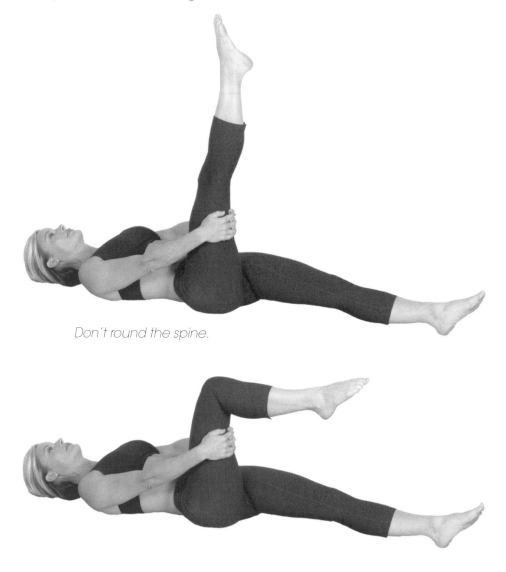

Don't round the spine.

Dynamic Seated Knee Kick

Hamstrings

Sit in a chair.

Start: Raise one leg and straighten the knee as much as comfortably possible.

Finish: Release the stretch by bending the knee and returning to the setup position.

Repeat as a continuous, controlled, fluid sequence 10 to 12 times.

Repeat on the other leg.

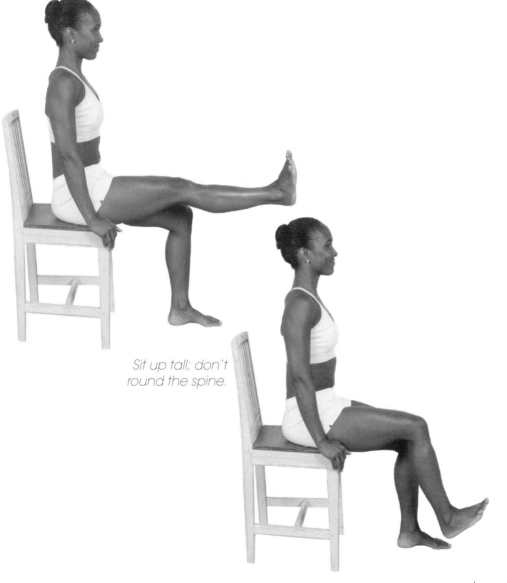

Sit up tall; don't round the spine.

CHAPTER 5

Calves, Shins, and Feet

In this chapter we'll do my favorite stretches for the lower legs and feet. Most of the impact forces on our body begin in these muscle groups, and they're forced to take on a great deal of mechanical stress for the rest of the body. As a result, these areas tend to require a great deal of attention to flexibility and mobility. All of us have had sore feet, calves, or shin splints at some time in our lives; these stretches reduce the incidence and severity of this type of stress. The stretches feel good and allow you to stay on your feet for longer periods of time.

CALVES

The calf is the generic name for the two muscles in the back of your lower leg—the gastrocnemius (upper calf) and the soleus (lower calf). The calves are used for pointing the toes and lifting the heels off the ground. They are also used explosively in any jumping activity, such as basketball or rope jumping. If you wear shoes with raised heels (such as high heels at the office), your calves are contracted a lot during the day and tend to be tight and inflexible. These stretches provide mobility around the ankle joint and keep your calves from getting too tight for your lower leg strength.

Static Heel Drop

Gastrocnemius

Place the ball of one foot on the edge of a step or curb. Push the heel down, keeping the knee straight. Place the other foot slightly in front.

Hold the stretch for 10 to 30 seconds.

Repeat on the other foot.

Hold onto something for balance, if necessary.

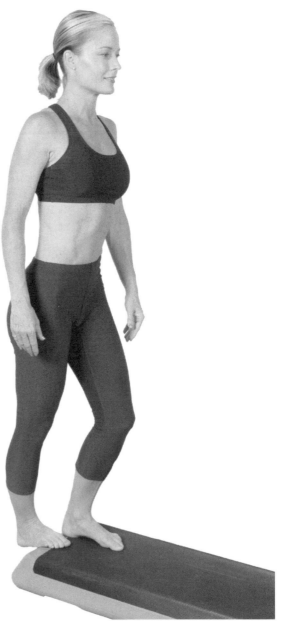

Static Heel Press

Gastrocnemius

Stand with one foot forward and one foot back, legs hip-width apart, feet facing forward. Bend the front knee and place the hands on the front thigh.

Hold the stretch for 10 to 30 seconds.

Repeat on the other leg.

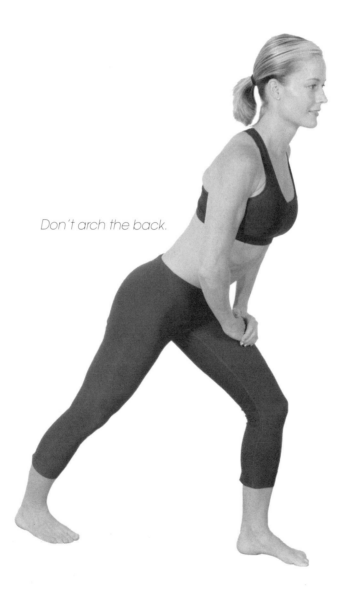

Don't arch the back.

Static Toe Up

Gastrocnemius

Stand with the ball of one foot on a curb or step and the other foot flat on the floor behind. Push the hips forward, keeping the knee straight.

Hold the stretch for 10 to 30 seconds.

Repeat on the other foot.

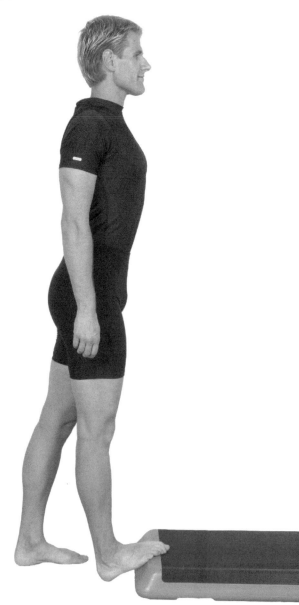

Static Seated Strap Foot Pull

Gastrocnemius

Extend the legs straight out in front. Place the strap around the ball of one foot. Use the strap to pull the foot closer to the body.

Hold the stretch for 10 to 30 seconds.

Repeat on the other leg.

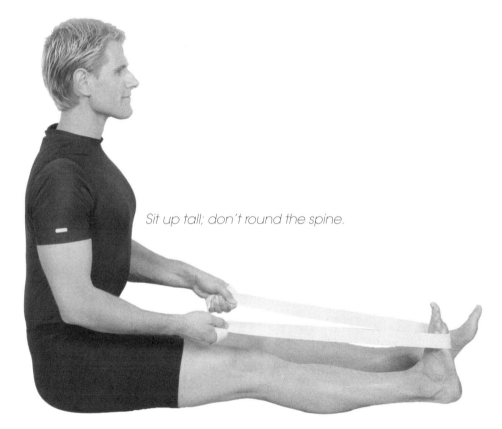

Sit up tall; don't round the spine.

Dynamic Seated Flex and Point

Gastrocnemius

Extend the legs straight out in front with knees very slightly bent.

Start: Flex feet toward the body.

Finish: Release the stretch by pointing the feet as far from the body as comfortably possible.

Sit up tall; don't round the spine.

Repeat as a continuous, controlled, fluid sequence 10 to 12 times.

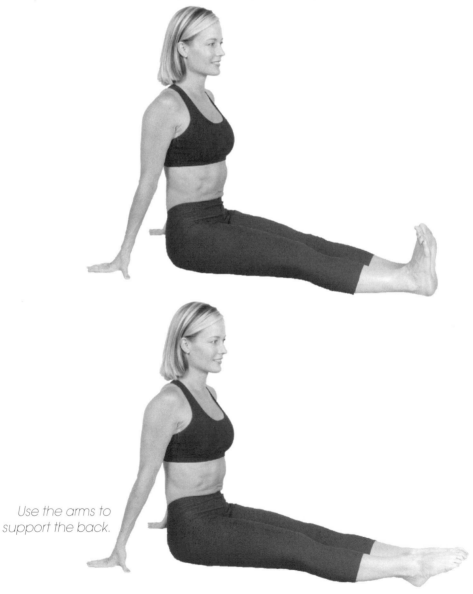

Use the arms to support the back.

Dynamic Heel Drop

Gastrocnemius

Place the ball of one foot on the edge of a step or curb. Place the other foot slightly in front.

Start: Lower the heel, keeping the knee straight.

Finish: Release the stretch by lifting the heel as high as comfortably possible.

Repeat as a continuous, controlled, fluid sequence 10 to 12 times.

Repeat on the other leg.

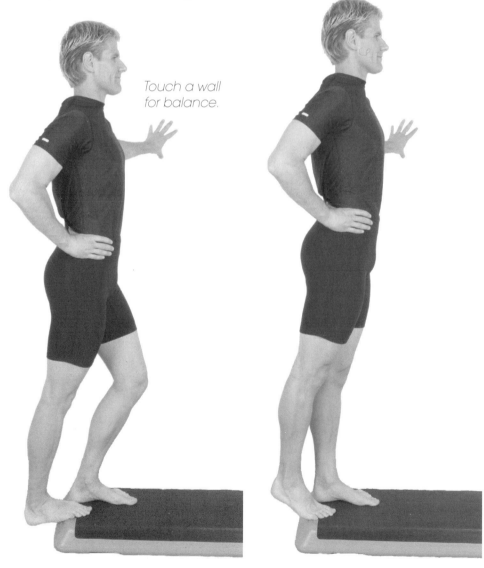

Touch a wall for balance.

Static Thinker Pose

Achilles tendon, soleus

Kneel down on one knee and sit back on the heel. Place the opposite foot next to the knee, keeping the heel on the floor.

Use the arms for balance.

Hold the stretch for 10 to 30 seconds.

Repeat on the other leg.

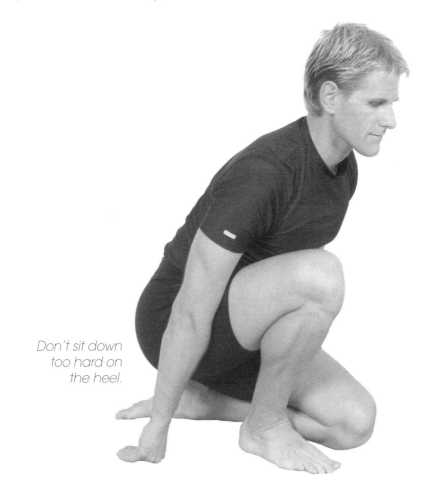

Don't sit down too hard on the heel.

Static Bent-Knee Heel Drop

Achilles tendon, soleus

Place the ball of one foot on the edge of a step or curb. Push the heel down, keeping the knee bent. Place the other foot in front.

Hold the stretch for 10 to 30 seconds.

Repeat on the other foot.

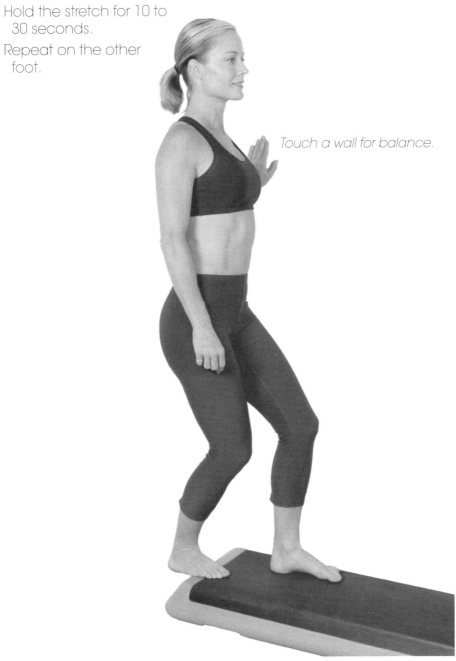

Touch a wall for balance.

Static Bent-Knee Heel Press

Achilles tendon, soleus

Place the feet in a split stance, hip-width apart and facing forward. Slide the back foot away from the body, keeping both knees bent.

Hold the stretch for 10 to 30 seconds.

Repeat on the other foot.

Touch a wall for balance, if necessary.

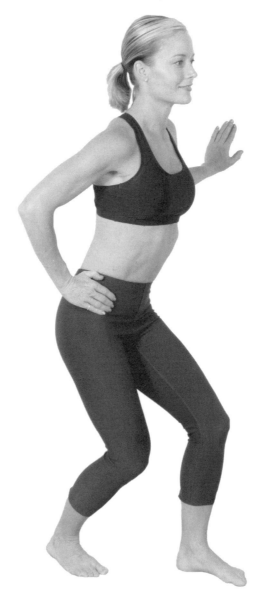

Dynamic Bent-Knee Heel Press

Achilles tendon, soleus

Stand with one foot forward and one foot back, hip-width apart and feet facing forward.

Start: Bend both knees and press the back heel toward the floor while keeping the back knee bent.

Finish: Release the stretch by straightening the back leg.

Repeat as a continuous, controlled, fluid sequence 10 to 12 times.

Repeat on the other leg.

Touch a wall or hold onto something for balance, if necessary.

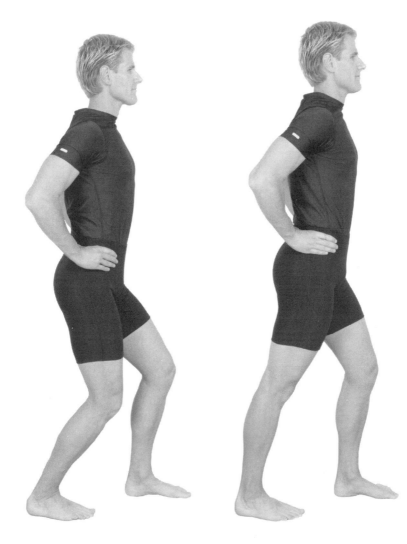

Dynamic Seated Bent-Knee Flex and Point

Achilles tendon, soleus

Extend the legs straight out in front with knees bent.

Start: Flex the feet toward you as far as comfortably possible, keeping the knees bent.

Finish: Release the stretch by flexing the foot as far away from the body as comfortably possible.

Repeat as a continuous, controlled, fluid sequence 10 to 12 times.

Use the arms as an anchor to support the back, if necessary.

Sit up tall; don't round the spine.

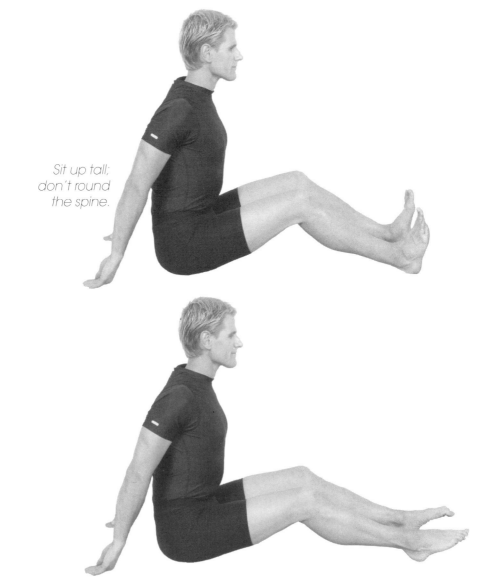

SHINS

The muscles of the shin work in partnership with the calves to flex and extend the ankle. The shin muscle is often overlooked in daily stretches, but flexible shins help in activities that use the calves. If we have flexible shin muscles, the toes can point farther and the calves can contract with more force, which helps with many sports and everyday activities (e.g., exploding upward for a dunk, reaching up to a high cupboard).

Static Toe Drop

Tibialis anterior

Place the top of one foot against the edge of a curb or step. Place the other foot in front. Press the back leg forward while pointing the toes.

Hold the stretch for 10 to 30 seconds.

Repeat on the other leg.

Touch a wall or hold onto something for balance, if necessary.

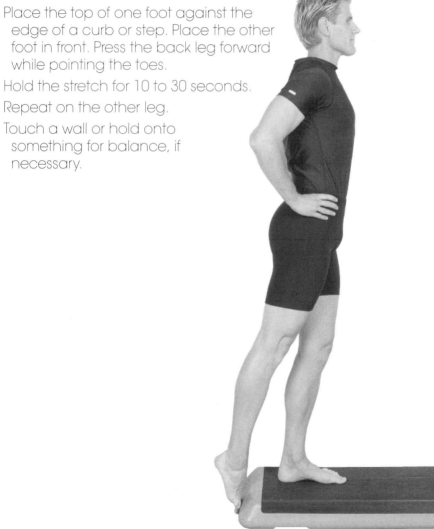

Static Seated Foot Pull

Tibialis anterior

Sit in a chair and rest one ankle just above the opposite knee. Pull the ball of the foot toward the body without twisting the ankle.

Hold the stretch for 10 to 30 seconds.

Repeat on the other leg.

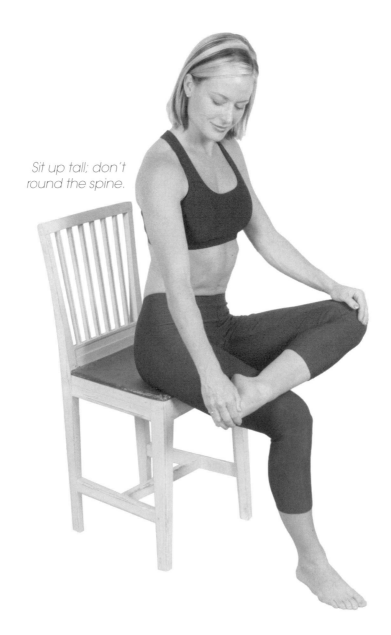

Sit up tall; don't round the spine.

Static Kneeling Toe Point and Sit

Tibialis anterior

Kneeling on the floor, point the toes and sit back directly on the heels.

Don't sit down too hard on the heels. Use the arms to support the upper body.

Hold the stretch for 10 to 30 seconds.

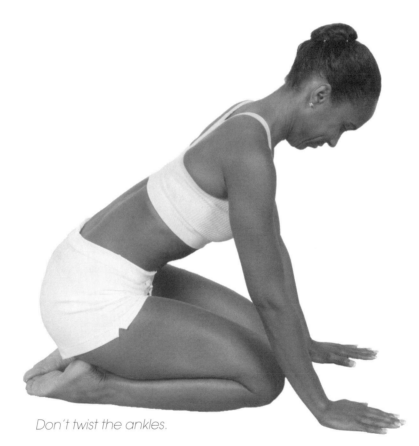

Don't twist the ankles.

Dynamic Seated Half-Circle

Tibialis anterior

Sit in a chair and rest one ankle just above the opposite knee.
Start: Point the foot.
Finish: Draw the shape of the lower half of a circle with the foot.
Repeat as a continuous, controlled, fluid sequence 10 to 12 times.
Repeat on the other leg.

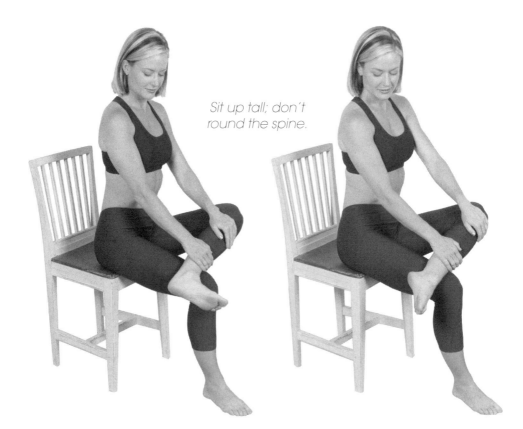

Sit up tall; don't round the spine.

FEET

Stretches for the feet feel good and help release much of the tension built up in the small muscles that support our whole body every time we take a step.

Dynamic Seated Ankle Pulls

Ankles

Sit in a chair and rest one ankle just above the opposite knee.

Start: Use a hand to move the sole of the foot inward.

Finish: Use a hand to move the sole of the foot outward.

Repeat as a continuous, controlled, fluid sequence 10 to 12 times.

Repeat on the other leg.

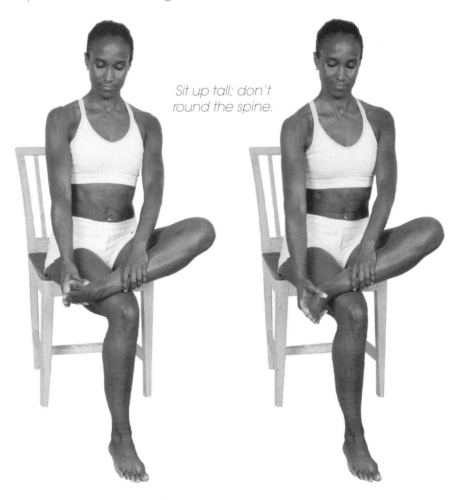

Sit up tall; don't round the spine.

Dynamic Seated Ankle Rolls

Ankles

Sit in a chair and rest one ankle just above the opposite knee.

Start: Point the foot.

Finish: Draw the shape of a large circle with the foot.

Repeat as a continuous, controlled, fluid sequence 10 to 12 times.

Repeat on the other leg.

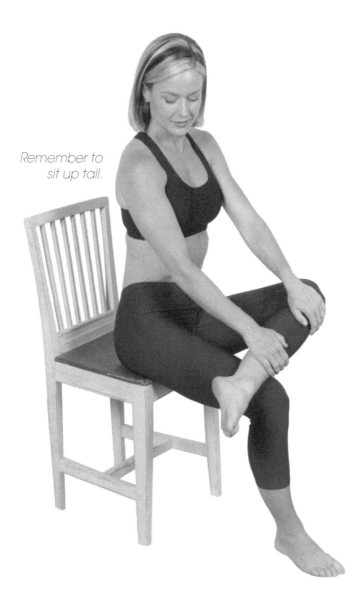

Remember to sit up tall.

Static Seated Foot Massage

Arch of foot

Sit in a chair and rest one ankle just above the opposite knee. Gently massage the arch of the foot with the hands. Gradually work deeper into the muscle under the arch.

Sit up tall; don't round the spine.

Repeat on the other foot.

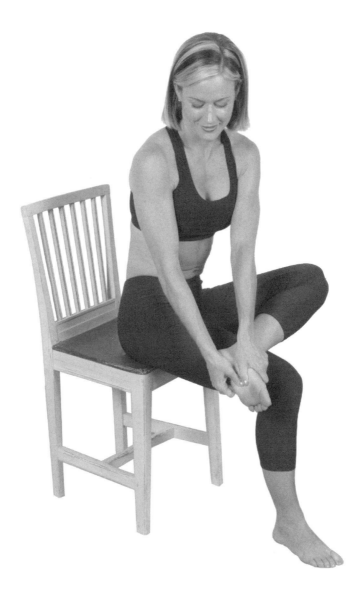

Dynamic Seated Toe Flex and Point

Arch of foot

Sit in a chair and rest one ankle just above the opposite knee.

Start: Point the toes down.

Finish: Flex the toes up.

Repeat as a continuous, controlled, fluid sequence 10 to 12 times.

Sit up tall; don't round the spine.

Repeat on the other foot.

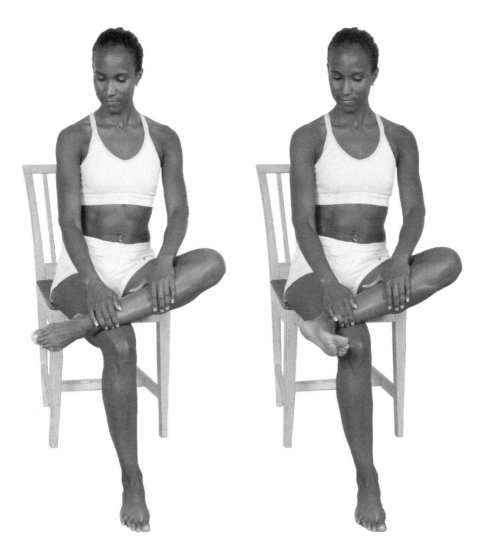

Static Seated Toe Pulls

Toes

Sit in a chair and rest one ankle just above the opposite knee.

Use a hand to pull the toes back toward the top of the foot.

Use the other hand to pull the toes down toward the sole of the foot.

Hold each stretch for 10 to 30 seconds.

Repeat on the other foot.

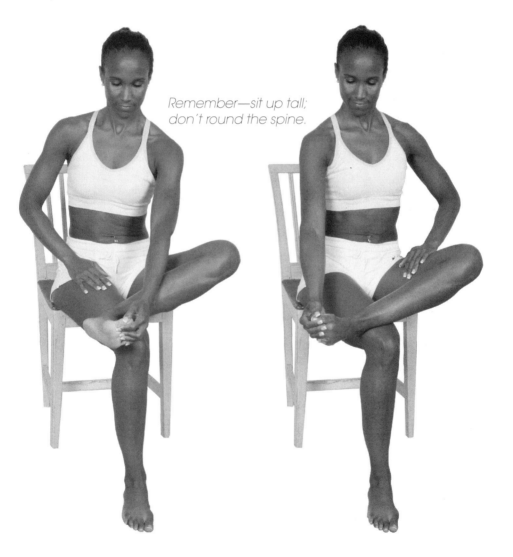

Remember—sit up tall; don't round the spine.

Dynamic Seated Toe Wiggle

Toes

Sit in a chair and rest one ankle just above the opposite knee.

Wiggle the toes as much as comfortably possible.

Repeat as a continuous, controlled, fluid sequence 10 to 12 times.

Remember to sit up tall and don't round the spine.

Repeat on the other foot.

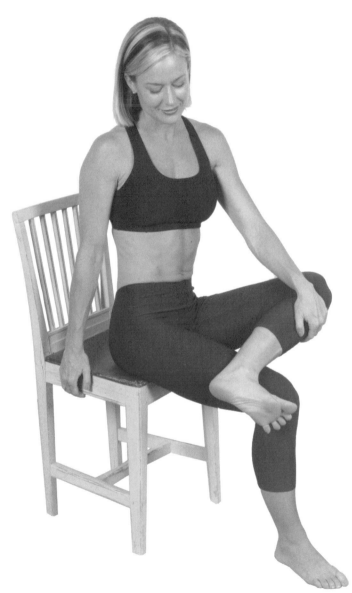

CHAPTER 6

Multiregion Stretches

In this chapter we'll focus on stretches that target multiple regions of the body at once. These stretches are more advanced and inspired by some of the world's most popular yoga poses. In addition to requiring good flexibility to execute these stretches, you'll find they take a great deal of strength to hold them in place. That is the beauty of these stretches. They energize the body while stretching some of the most important muscle groups at the same time. You might find it challenging to get into some of these stretch positions. I know I do. Don't get discouraged if you don't do the stretches perfectly right away. Take your time; be patient with yourself. You'll find that the stretches get easier each time you do them—and you won't believe how much stronger you'll become.

Lying Spinal Twist

Gluteals, trunk extensors, pectoralis

Begin by lying down with knees bent and palms together in front
of the chest. Straighten the arms toward the ceiling and let the
body fall to one side. Place the opposite arm up and over the
head to the floor behind. Turn the head to face the hand.

Hold the stretch for 10 to 30 seconds.

Repeat on the other side.

ASSISTED STRETCH

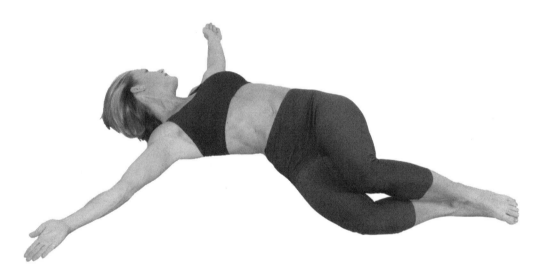

Triangle

Adductors, thoracic-lumbar rotators, trunk extensors

Stand with feet about three feet apart with one foot pointed forward and the other turned out about 90 degrees. Bend toward the turned-out foot and stretch the upper arm up over the head. Rest the lower hand on the ankle or calf. Turn the head to look up to the ceiling.

Hold the stretch for 10 to 30 seconds.

Repeat on the other side.

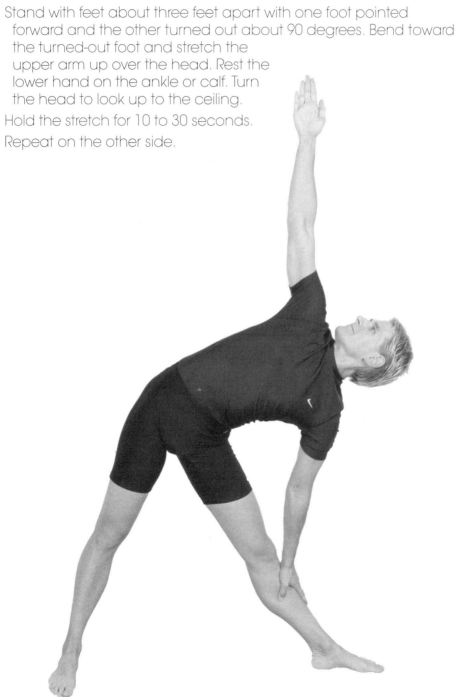

Extended Angle

Adductors, lateral trunk flexors, trunk extensors

Stand with feet about four feet apart with one foot pointed forward and the other turned out about 90 degrees. Bend the knee of the turned-out foot and lean toward the same foot. Stretch the upper arm up over the head so that it forms a straight line with the torso and leg; rest the lower arm on the thigh. Turn the head to look up to the ceiling.

Hold the stretch for 10 to 30 seconds.

Repeat on the other side.

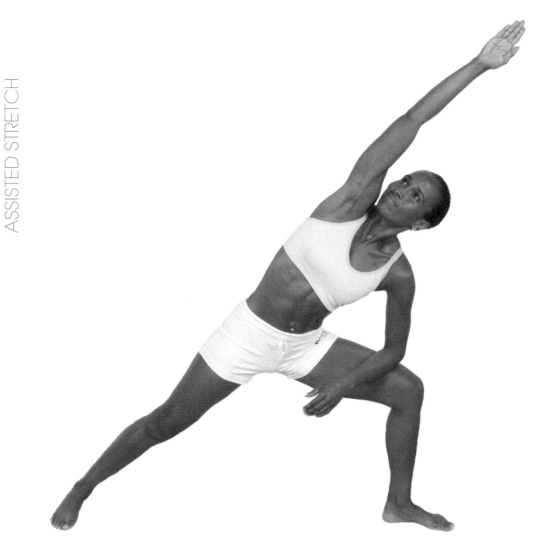

Warrior

Abdominals, hip flexors, gluteals

Stand with feet about four feet apart with one foot pointed forward and the other extended behind and turned out about 90 degrees. Bend the knee of the turned-out foot to 90 degrees. Raise both arms overhead with palms facing each other; rotate the upper body to face the direction of the bent knee.

Hold the stretch for 10 to 30 seconds.

Repeat on the other side.

Keep the back foot firmly planted and the back leg straight.

Chair

Achilles tendon, soleus, gluteals, abdominals

Stand with feet slightly apart. Bend the knees and lean the upper body forward slightly. Drop the hips as if sitting in a chair.

Keep palms slightly apart.

Hold the stretch for 10 to 30 seconds.

ASSISTED STRETCH

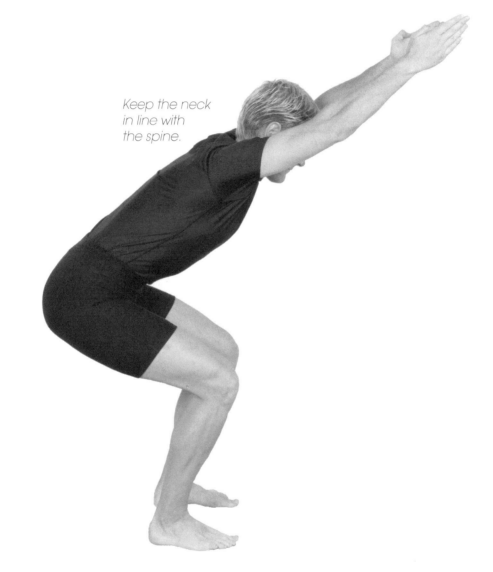

Keep the neck in line with the spine.

Downward-Facing Dog

Gastrocnemius, soleus, hamstrings, abdominals, pectoralis

Kneel with hands on the floor. Lift the tailbone and bring the knees off the floor. Bring the shoulders and head down. Keep the knees bent at first, then slowly bring the heels to the floor and straighten the knees.

Hold the stretch for 10 to 30 seconds.

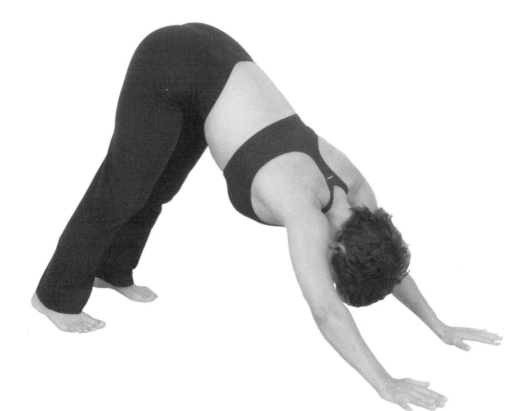

Upward-Facing Dog

Tibialis anterior, hip flexors, abdominals

Lie on the floor face down with the hands near the shoulders. Lift the body off the floor by pushing with the hands.

Don't extend beyond comfort for the lower back.

Hold the stretch for 10 to 30 seconds.

ASSISTED STRETCH

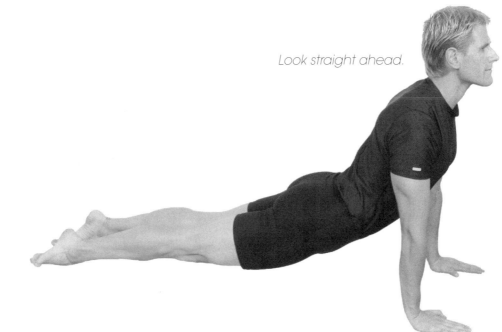

Look straight ahead.

Child's Pose

Tibialis anterior, quadriceps, trunk extensors, trapezius, rhomboids

From a kneeling position, sit back on the heels, then bring the forehead to the floor. Rest the arms alongside the body with palms facing up.

Hold the stretch for 10 to 30 seconds.

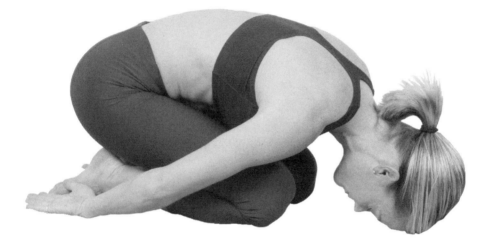

Forward Bend

Hamstrings, trunk extensors

Stand with feet together and raise the arms overhead. Bend forward at the hips and bring the nose toward the knees and hands to (or toward) the floor.

Hold the stretch for 10 to 30 seconds.

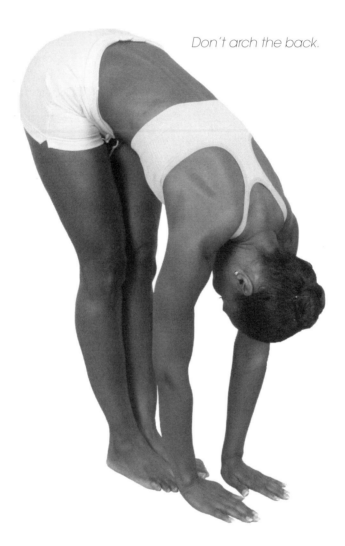

Don't arch the back.

Reverse Prayer

Wrists, deltoid (front shoulder)

Stand with feet comfortably apart and arms beside the body. Pull the shoulders back and place the backs of the hands together. Slide the hands as far up the spine as comfortably possible with the fingers pointing to the ceiling. Pull the shoulders back.

Hold the stretch for 10 to 30 seconds.

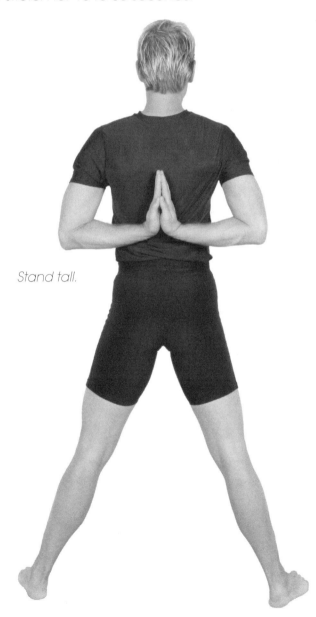

Stand tall.

Fan

Hamstrings, adductors, trunk extensors

Stand with feet three to four feet apart with feet facing forward. Bend forward at the hips and place the hands on the floor in front of the feet.

Hold the stretch for 10 to 30 seconds.

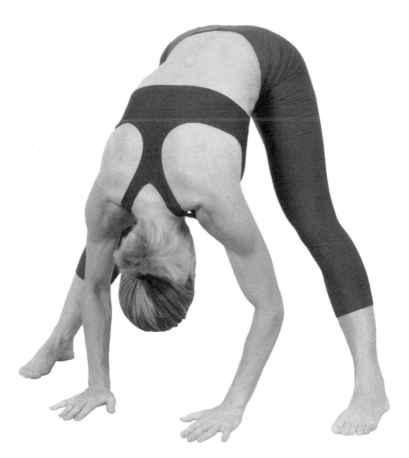

Sitting Angular Leg Extension

Hamstrings, adductors, trunk extensors

Sit on the floor and spread the legs apart as far as comfortably possible. Bend forward at the hip and reach toward the ankle with both arms.

Hold the stretch for 10 to 30 seconds.

Repeat on the other side.

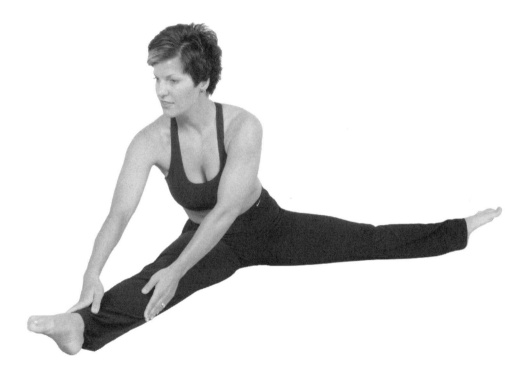

Dynamic Four-Legged Table

Biceps, hip flexors, deltoids, wrist extensors

Seated on the floor, extend the legs straight out in front with knees bent. Keep the feet hip-width apart. Place the hands behind, with fingers facing forward.

Start: Lift the hips off the floor and try to place the knees, hips, and shoulders parallel to the floor. Keep the head in line with the spine, looking up.

Finish: Release the stretch by returning to seated position.

Repeat as a continuous, controlled, fluid sequence 10 to 12 times.

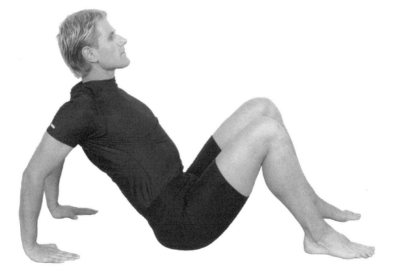

Keep the knees over the ankles and the shoulders over the hands.

Static Reverse Plank

Deltoids, wrists, biceps

Seated on the floor, extend the legs straight out in front. Place the hands behind with fingers facing forward. Keep the legs straight and lift the hips off the floor. The knees, hips, and shoulders should be in a straight line. Keep the head in line with the spine.

Hold the stretch for 10 to 30 seconds.

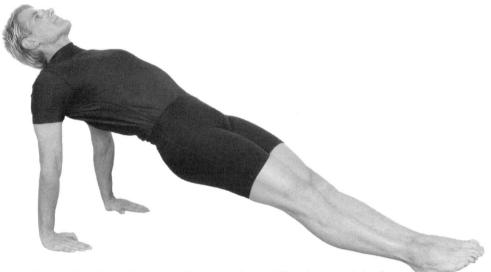

Keep the shoulders over the hands and the toes pointed.

PART II

Fitness and Sports Routines

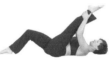
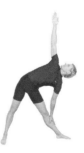

CHAPTER 7

Fitness Routines

The routines in this chapter are organized in a way that makes it easy for you to get a good stretch workout whenever you want one; the stretches flow smoothly and easily from one to another. You can do the routine in as little as 10 minutes or take as long as 40 minutes.

For convenience, I've included a small photo of each stretch in the routine. If you have trouble recalling how to do a particular stretch in a routine, simply turn back to part I for a review of the stretch.

You are in charge. If you don't like one of the stretches in a routine, feel free to substitute it with another stretch for the same muscle group. Don't get comfortable with just one routine. Mix them up; try a different one every day. There are 13 routines in part II—more than enough to take you through every day of the week.

10-MINUTE TOTAL BODY ROUTINE

Approximate time: 10 minutes

This is the perfect routine if you want to stretch your whole body but don't have a lot of time. Nothing fancy in this routine—just simple stretches, all from a standing position, designed to target all the most important muscle groups in a minimum amount of time.

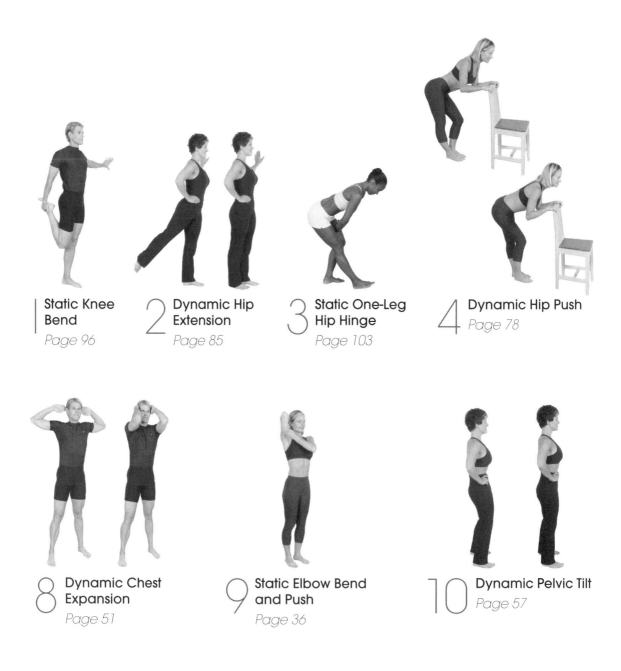

1 Static Knee Bend
Page 96

2 Dynamic Hip Extension
Page 85

3 Static One-Leg Hip Hinge
Page 103

4 Dynamic Hip Push
Page 78

8 Dynamic Chest Expansion
Page 51

9 Static Elbow Bend and Push
Page 36

10 Dynamic Pelvic Tilt
Page 57

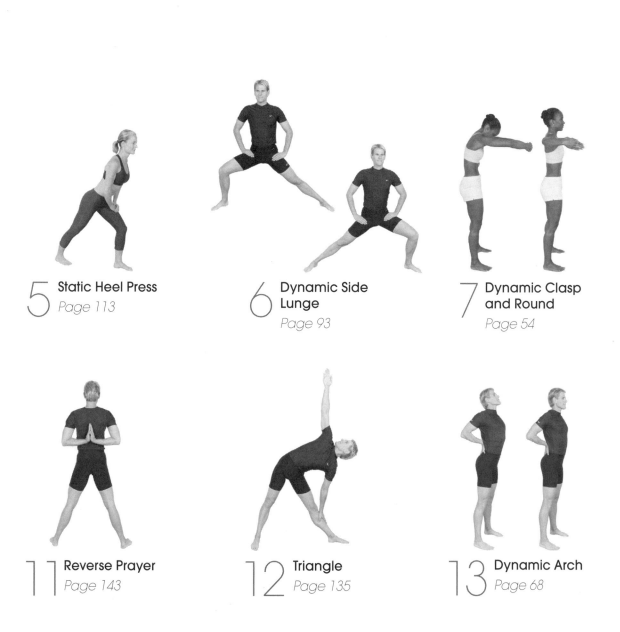

5 **Static Heel Press**
Page 113

6 **Dynamic Side Lunge**
Page 93

7 **Dynamic Clasp and Round**
Page 54

11 **Reverse Prayer**
Page 143

12 **Triangle**
Page 135

13 **Dynamic Arch**
Page 68

20-MINUTE TOTAL BODY ROUTINE

Approximate time: 20 minutes

This routine is perfect if you have more than 10 minutes but not enough time to do the 40-minute stretch routine. This routine takes you through sitting and lying-down stretches first, and then finishes with standing stretches. Although this routine doesn't take a lot of time, it has several stretches that will challenge you much more than the 10-minute routine does. This is a power-packed routine filled with flowing sequences that will balance your body from head to toe.

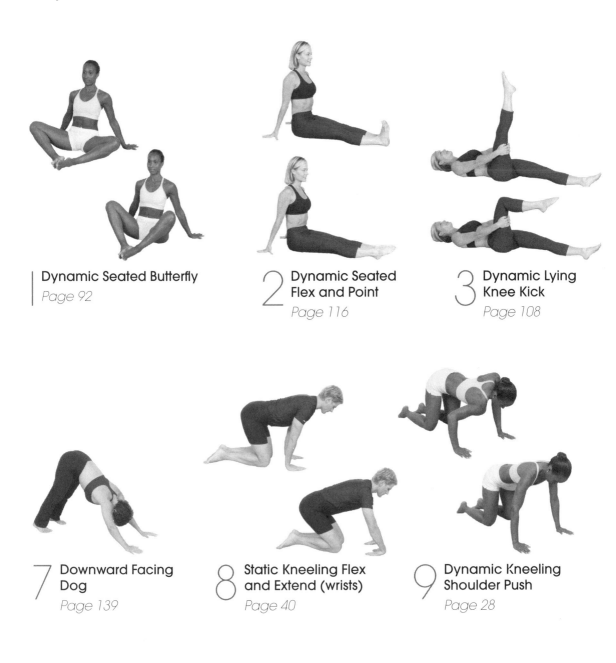

1 Dynamic Seated Butterfly
Page 92

2 Dynamic Seated Flex and Point
Page 116

3 Dynamic Lying Knee Kick
Page 108

7 Downward Facing Dog
Page 139

8 Static Kneeling Flex and Extend (wrists)
Page 40

9 Dynamic Kneeling Shoulder Push
Page 28

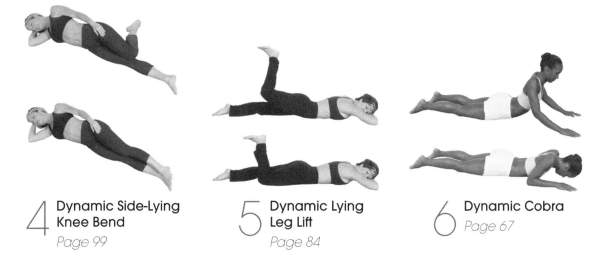

4 **Dynamic Side-Lying Knee Bend**
Page 99

5 **Dynamic Lying Leg Lift**
Page 84

6 **Dynamic Cobra**
Page 67

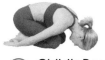

10 **Child's Pose**
Page 141

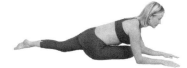

11 **Static Dancer**
Page 73

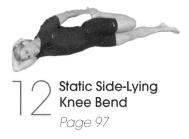

12 **Static Side-Lying Knee Bend**
Page 97

(continued)

(continued)

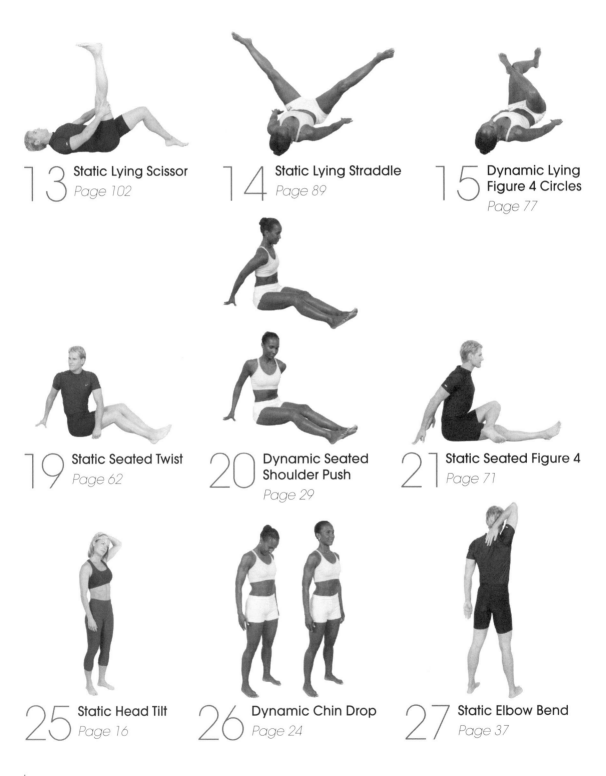

13 **Static Lying Scissor**
Page 102

14 **Static Lying Straddle**
Page 89

15 **Dynamic Lying Figure 4 Circles**
Page 77

19 **Static Seated Twist**
Page 62

20 **Dynamic Seated Shoulder Push**
Page 29

21 **Static Seated Figure 4**
Page 71

25 **Static Head Tilt**
Page 16

26 **Dynamic Chin Drop**
Page 24

27 **Static Elbow Bend**
Page 37

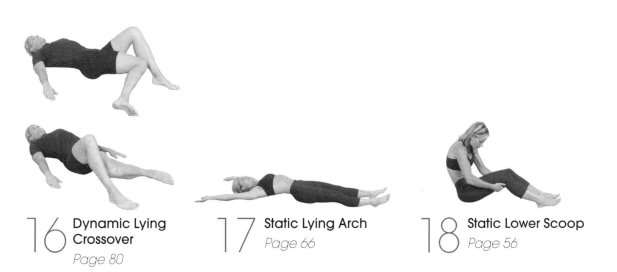

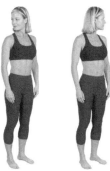

16 Dynamic Lying Crossover
Page 80

17 Static Lying Arch
Page 66

18 Static Lower Scoop
Page 56

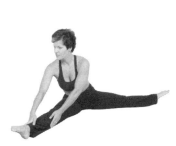

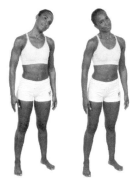

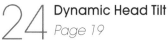

22 Sitting Angular Leg Extension
Page 145

23 Dynamic Head Turn
Page 20

24 Dynamic Head Tilt
Page 19

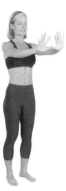

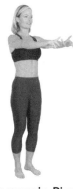

28 Dynamic Web Hands
Page 46

29 Dynamic Piano Fingers
Page 45

40-MINUTE TOTAL BODY ROUTINE

Approximate time: 40 minutes

This is the most challenging and comprehensive routine in this book and should be done when you have enough time and when you feel your body needs a complete and thorough stretch release. This routine is inspired by sequences you might see in a typical yoga class and is great preparation (if you have never taken yoga) or substitution (if you don't have time to go to a class) for yoga. You begin this routine standing, work your way to the floor gradually, and move back up to standing at the end of the routine. You'll notice that about 30 minutes into the routine you'll need a chair to execute some of the stretches. If you would like to shorten the routine to 30 minutes, this is a good place to stop; if you're ready to complete the routine, then grab a chair and continue. Be prepared to feel strong, stretched, and centered when you finish this routine.

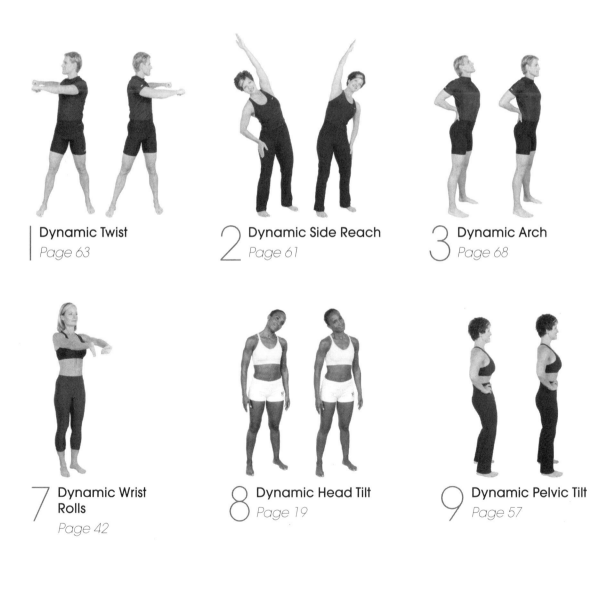

1 **Dynamic Twist**
Page 63

2 **Dynamic Side Reach**
Page 61

3 **Dynamic Arch**
Page 68

7 **Dynamic Wrist Rolls**
Page 42

8 **Dynamic Head Tilt**
Page 19

9 **Dynamic Pelvic Tilt**
Page 57

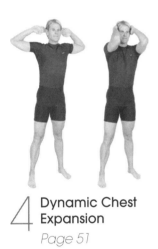

4 Dynamic Chest
Expansion
Page 51

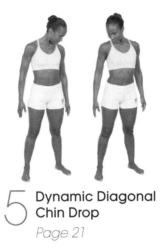

5 Dynamic Diagonal
Chin Drop
Page 21

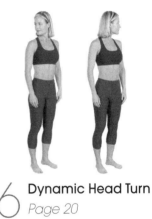

6 Dynamic Head Turn
Page 20

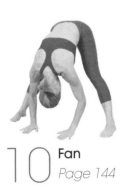

10 Fan
Page 144

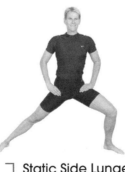

11 Static Side Lunge
Page 87

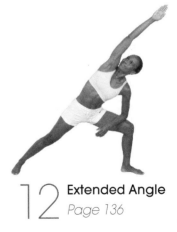

12 Extended Angle
Page 136

(continued)

40-MINUTE TOTAL BODY ROUTINE

(continued)

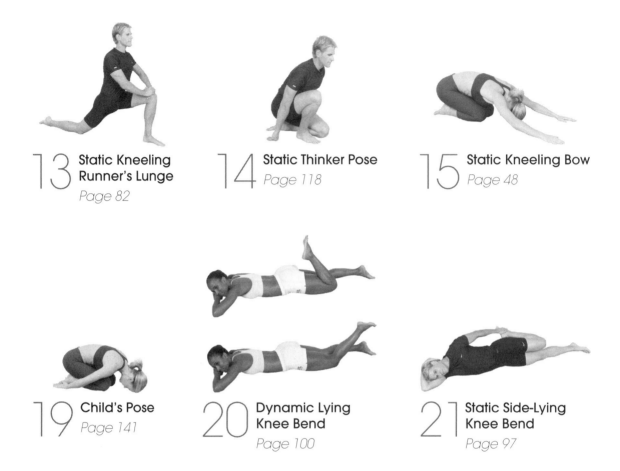

13 **Static Kneeling Runner's Lunge**
Page 82

14 **Static Thinker Pose**
Page 118

15 **Static Kneeling Bow**
Page 48

19 **Child's Pose**
Page 141

20 **Dynamic Lying Knee Bend**
Page 100

21 **Static Side-Lying Knee Bend**
Page 97

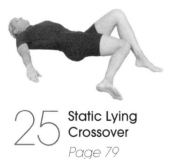

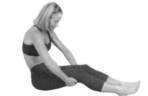

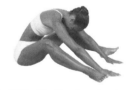

25 **Static Lying Crossover**
Page 79

26 **Static Upper Scoop**
Page 53

27 **Static Seated Forward Bend**
Page 55

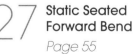

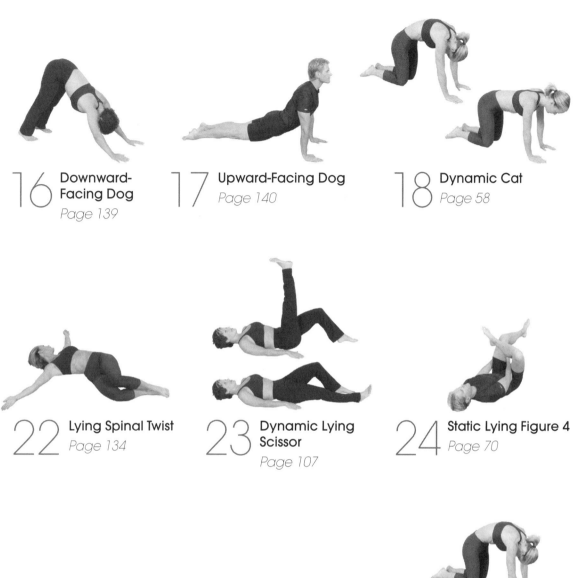

16 **Downward-Facing Dog**
Page 139

17 **Upward-Facing Dog**
Page 140

18 **Dynamic Cat**
Page 58

22 **Lying Spinal Twist**
Page 134

23 **Dynamic Lying Scissor**
Page 107

24 **Static Lying Figure 4**
Page 70

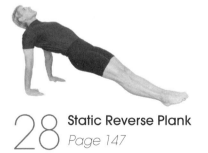

28 **Static Reverse Plank**
Page 147

29 **Static Lower Scoop**
Page 56

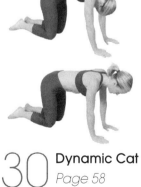

30 **Dynamic Cat**
Page 58

(continued)

40-MINUTE TOTAL BODY ROUTINE

(continued)

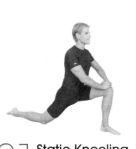

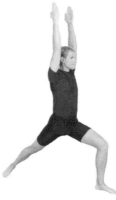

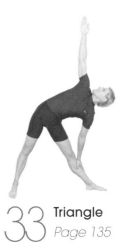

31 **Static Kneeling Runner's Lunge**
Page 82

32 **Warrior**
Page 137

33 **Triangle**
Page 135

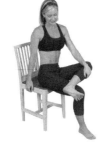

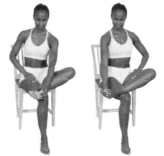

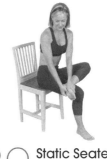

37 **Dynamic Seated Toe Wiggle**
Page 132

38 **Static Seated Toe Pulls**
Page 131

39 **Static Seated Foot Massage**
Page 129

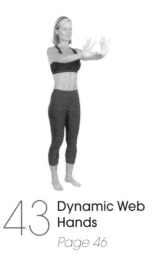

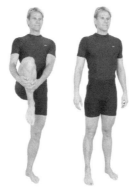

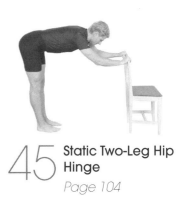

43 **Dynamic Web Hands**
Page 46

44 **Dynamic Knee Hug**
Page 76

45 **Static Two-Leg Hip Hinge**
Page 104

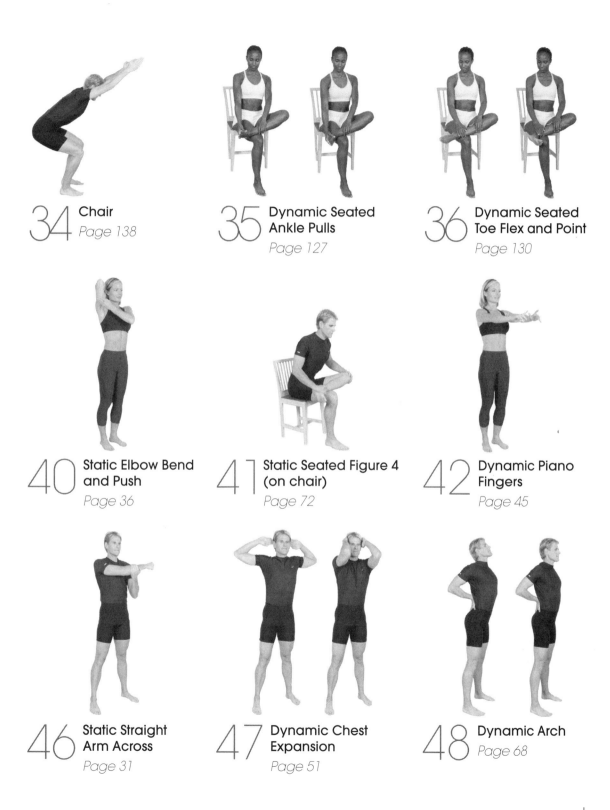

34 Chair
Page 138

35 Dynamic Seated Ankle Pulls
Page 127

36 Dynamic Seated Toe Flex and Point
Page 130

40 Static Elbow Bend and Push
Page 36

41 Static Seated Figure 4 (on chair)
Page 72

42 Dynamic Piano Fingers
Page 45

46 Static Straight Arm Across
Page 31

47 Dynamic Chest Expansion
Page 51

48 Dynamic Arch
Page 68

CHAPTER 8

Sports Routines

This chapter presents three stretch routines for a range of sports. The sports are grouped into three categories: (1) swinging and throwing sports, (2) endurance and distance sports, and (3) power and jumping sports. In each category I have tried to include the most popular sports as well as several others that are more obscure or unusual. I hope you'll find your favorite sport in one of the categories. Each sequence of stretches is designed to provide flexibility and strength appropriate for the sports included in that category. For example, there are many stretches for the shoulder and back in the swinging and throwing category. Each routine is designed to improve the range of motion in the joints that are active when playing the sport and to release the tension in the muscles that tend to be overworked or stressed through participation in the sport.

SWINGING AND THROWING SPORTS

Tennis, squash, racquetball, badminton, table tennis, golf, baseball, softball, cricket, curling, water polo, bowling

Approximate time: 30 minutes

Swinging and throwing sports typically emphasize the upper body during activity. This doesn't mean the lower body is not important in the activity but that flexibility and strength of the upper body is most critical. In swinging and throwing sports, the muscles of the neck, shoulders, arms, and torso are continually challenged and require a great deal of mobility. This stretch routine is the perfect complement for these activities.

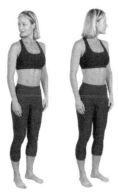

Dynamic Head Turn
Page 20

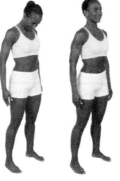

2 **Dynamic Chin Drop**
Page 24

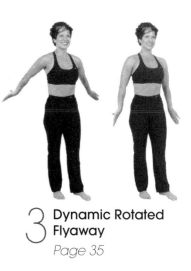

3 **Dynamic Rotated Flyaway**
Page 35

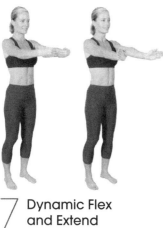

7 **Dynamic Flex and Extend**
Page 41

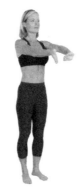

8 **Dynamic Wrist Rolls**
Page 42

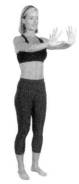

9 **Dynamic Web Hands**
Page 46

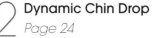

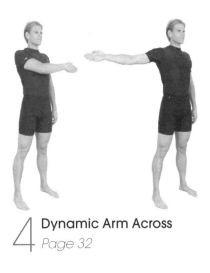

4 **Dynamic Arm Across**
Page 32

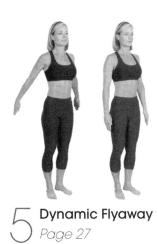

5 **Dynamic Flyaway**
Page 27

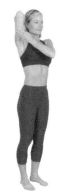

6 **Static Elbow Bend and Push**
Page 36

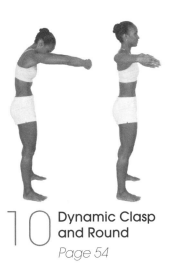

10 **Dynamic Clasp and Round**
Page 54

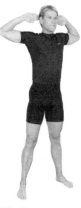

11 **Static Chest Expansion**
Page 50

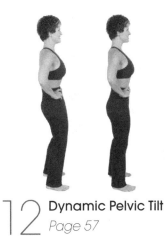

12 **Dynamic Pelvic Tilt**
Page 57

(continued)

SWINGING AND THROWING SPORTS

(continued)

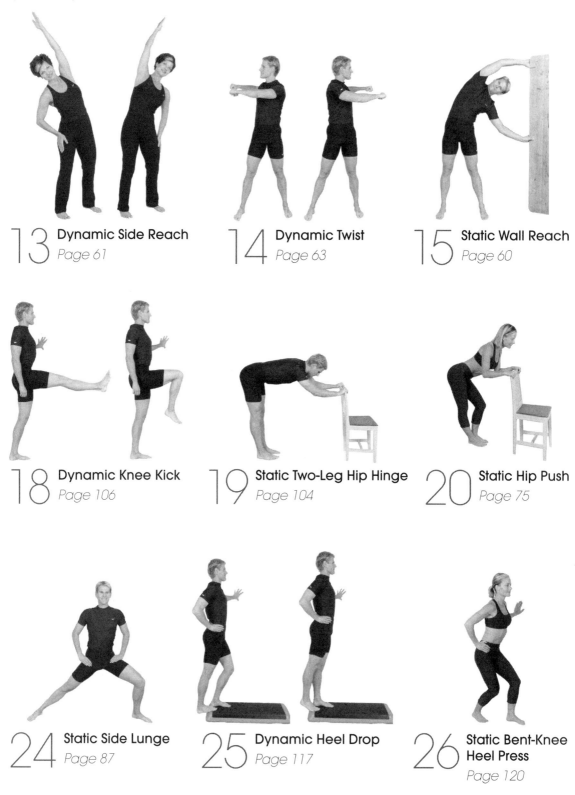

13 **Dynamic Side Reach**
Page 61

14 **Dynamic Twist**
Page 63

15 **Static Wall Reach**
Page 60

18 **Dynamic Knee Kick**
Page 106

19 **Static Two-Leg Hip Hinge**
Page 104

20 **Static Hip Push**
Page 75

24 **Static Side Lunge**
Page 87

25 **Dynamic Heel Drop**
Page 117

26 **Static Bent-Knee Heel Press**
Page 120

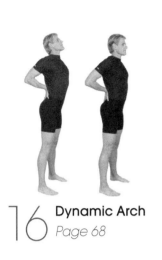

16 **Dynamic Arch**
Page 68

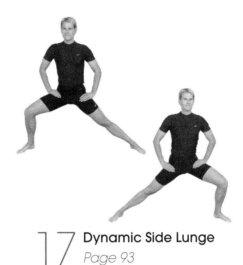

17 **Dynamic Side Lunge**
Page 93

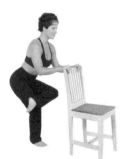

21 **Static Figure 4**
Page 74

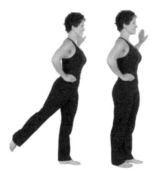

22 **Dynamic Hip Extension**
Page 85

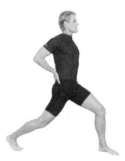

23 **Static Lunge**
Page 81

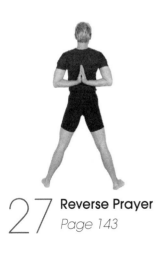

27 **Reverse Prayer**
Page 143

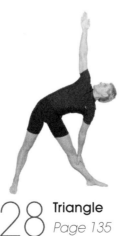

28 **Triangle**
Page 135

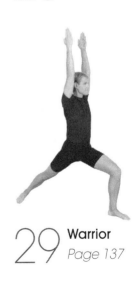

29 **Warrior**
Page 137

ENDURANCE AND DISTANCE SPORTS

Running, walking, cross-country skiing, cycling, field hockey, rowing, soccer, kayaking, lacrosse, rock climbing, Australian rules football, swimming

Approximate time: 30 minutes

In endurance and distance sports the key factor is sustaining the activity over time, usually with an emphasis on the lower body muscles. Grouping soccer and rock climbing into the same category might seem strange, but both activities require continued muscular activity over a long time as well as great power and strength from the lower body. This routine makes all endurance and distance sports easier to do and reduces recovery time between events or contests.

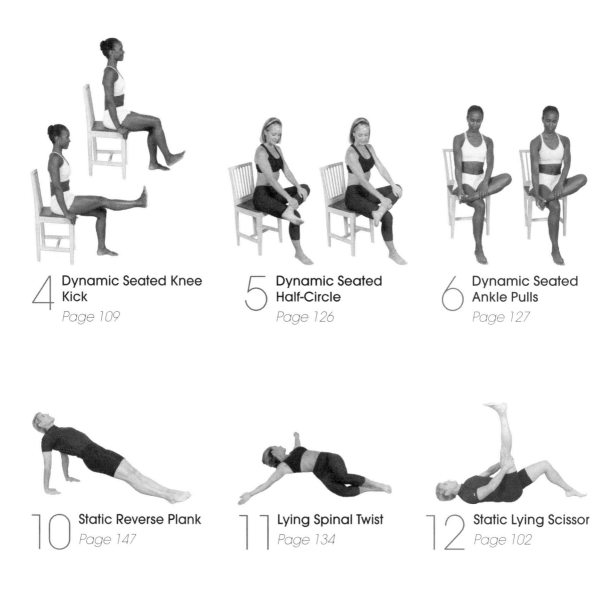

4 **Dynamic Seated Knee Kick**
Page 109

5 **Dynamic Seated Half-Circle**
Page 126

6 **Dynamic Seated Ankle Pulls**
Page 127

10 **Static Reverse Plank** *Page 147*

11 **Lying Spinal Twist** *Page 134*

12 **Static Lying Scissor** *Page 102*

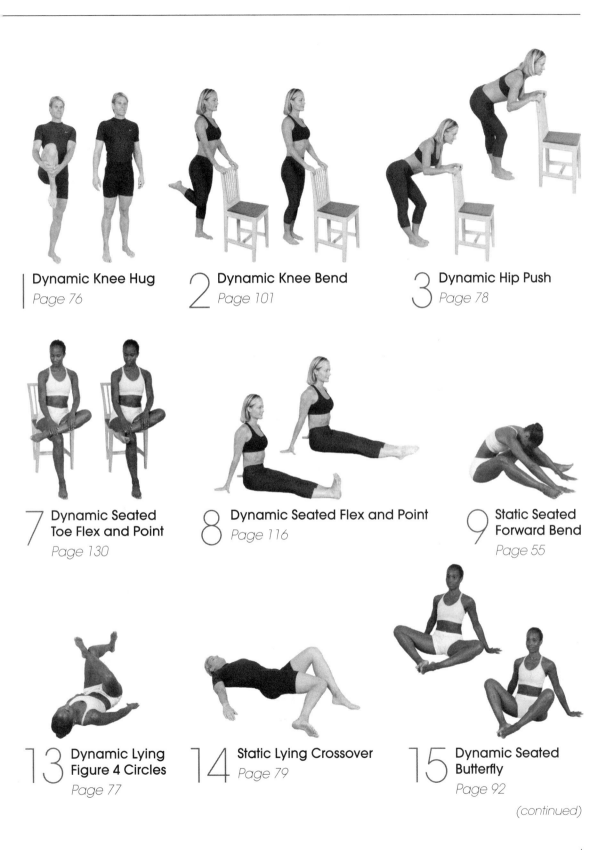

Dynamic Knee Hug
Page 76

2 **Dynamic Knee Bend**
Page 101

3 **Dynamic Hip Push**
Page 78

7 **Dynamic Seated Toe Flex and Point**
Page 130

8 **Dynamic Seated Flex and Point**
Page 116

9 **Static Seated Forward Bend**
Page 55

13 **Dynamic Lying Figure 4 Circles**
Page 77

14 **Static Lying Crossover**
Page 79

15 **Dynamic Seated Butterfly**
Page 92

(continued)

ENDURANCE AND DISTANCE SPORTS

(continued)

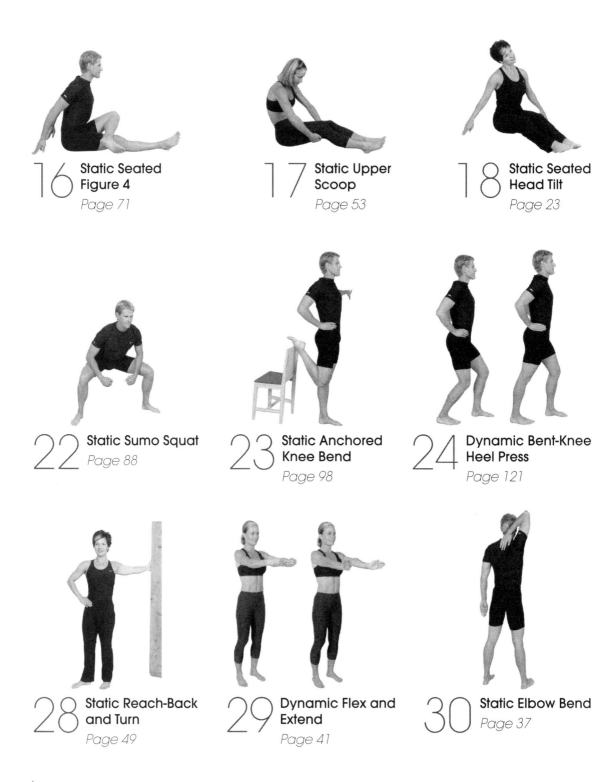

16 **Static Seated Figure 4**
Page 71

17 **Static Upper Scoop**
Page 53

18 **Static Seated Head Tilt**
Page 23

22 **Static Sumo Squat**
Page 88

23 **Static Anchored Knee Bend**
Page 98

24 **Dynamic Bent-Knee Heel Press**
Page 121

28 **Static Reach-Back and Turn**
Page 49

29 **Dynamic Flex and Extend**
Page 41

30 **Static Elbow Bend**
Page 37

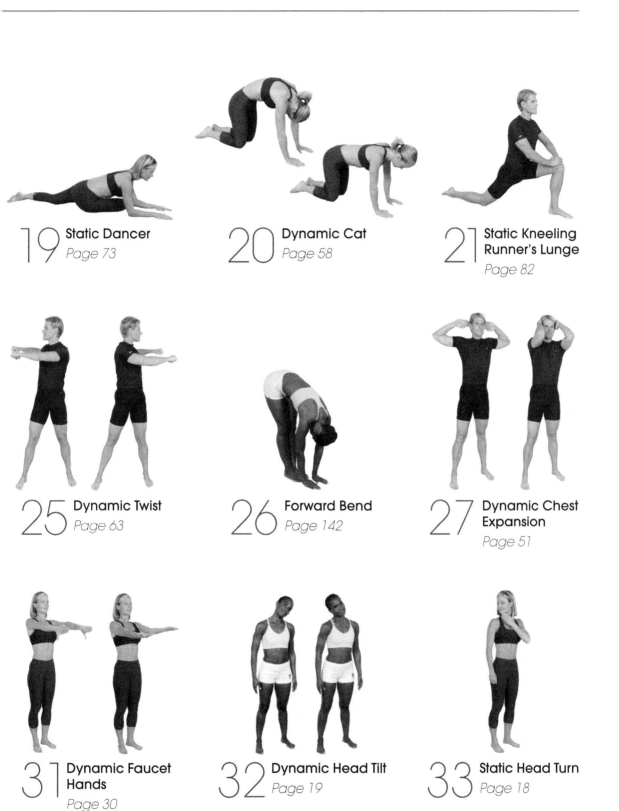

19 Static Dancer
Page 73

20 Dynamic Cat
Page 58

21 Static Kneeling Runner's Lunge
Page 82

25 Dynamic Twist
Page 63

26 Forward Bend
Page 142

27 Dynamic Chest Expansion
Page 51

31 Dynamic Faucet Hands
Page 30

32 Dynamic Head Tilt
Page 19

33 Static Head Turn
Page 18

POWER AND JUMPING SPORTS

Boxing, wrestling, martial arts, basketball, volleyball, football, rugby, ice hockey, netball, gymnastics, figure skating, surfing, snowboarding, snow skiing, water skiing

Approximate time: 30 minutes

All power and jumping sports require explosive force and strength. Whether you're kicking in karate, tumbling in gymnastics, or jumping in basketball, these sports require the muscles to fire quickly and powerfully, usually in short bursts rather than in long sustained effort. The power and jumping sequence helps you build the mobility you need to perform these sports and reduce the risk of injury along the way.

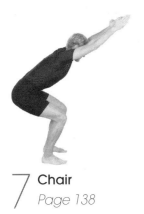

Dynamic Head Tilt
Page 19

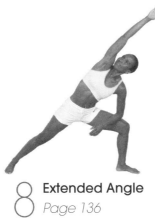

Dynamic Head Turn
Page 20

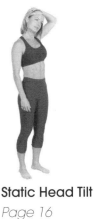

Static Head Tilt
Page 16

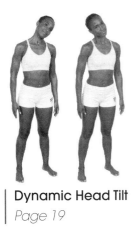

7 **Chair**
Page 138

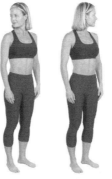

8 **Extended Angle**
Page 136

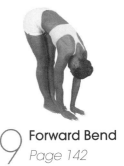

9 **Forward Bend**
Page 142

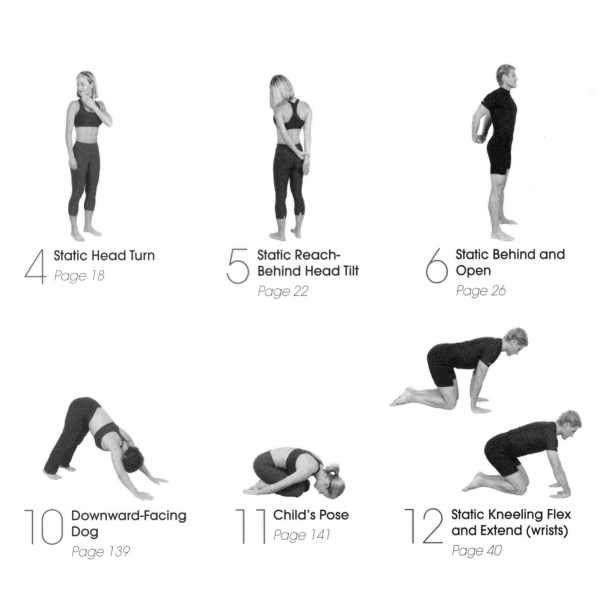

4 Static Head Turn
Page 18

5 Static Reach-
Behind Head Tilt
Page 22

6 Static Behind and
Open
Page 26

10 Downward-Facing
Dog
Page 139

11 Child's Pose
Page 141

12 Static Kneeling Flex
and Extend (wrists)
Page 40

(continued)

POWER AND JUMPING SPORTS

(continued)

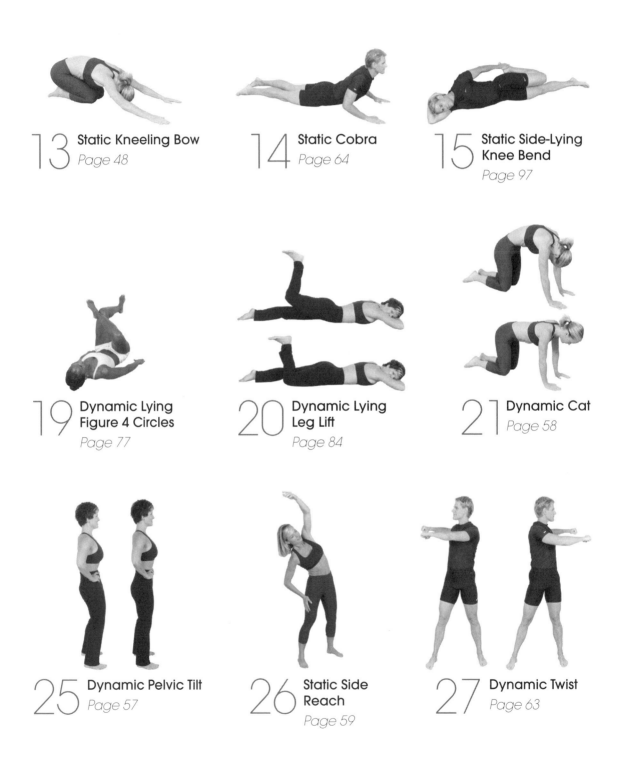

13 **Static Kneeling Bow**
Page 48

14 **Static Cobra**
Page 64

15 **Static Side-Lying Knee Bend**
Page 97

19 **Dynamic Lying Figure 4 Circles**
Page 77

20 **Dynamic Lying Leg Lift**
Page 84

21 **Dynamic Cat**
Page 58

25 **Dynamic Pelvic Tilt**
Page 57

26 **Static Side Reach**
Page 59

27 **Dynamic Twist**
Page 63

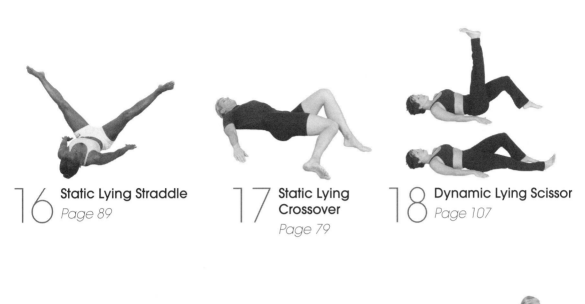

16 **Static Lying Straddle**
Page 89

17 **Static Lying Crossover**
Page 79

18 **Dynamic Lying Scissor**
Page 107

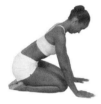

22 **Static Kneeling Toe Point and Sit**
Page 125

23 **Static Thinker Pose**
Page 118

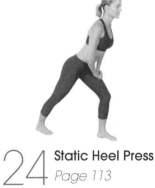

24 **Static Heel Press**
Page 113

28 **Fan**
Page 144

CHAPTER 9

Specialty Stretch Routines

In this chapter, each routine has a theme. One is designed to help wake you up in the morning. Another helps you relax before you go to bed at night. Others help with lower back problems, tight shoulders and neck, upper body and lower body, and everyday bending, reaching, and playing. I love these routines because they fit so conveniently into life. It's easy to make time for a few minutes' worth of stretching. And the payoffs are immediate and real. The routines make you feel better, more relaxed, as you progress through the day; they also prepare you for the next day to come. They are my favorites—I hope they work for you, too.

MORNING STRETCH ROUTINE

Approximate time: 10 minutes

This routine moves you from a seated position to standing, so you can literally do it from the edge of your bed when you first wake up in the morning. You'll notice this routine uses simple stretches for the most part to help you begin your day with an energizing start.

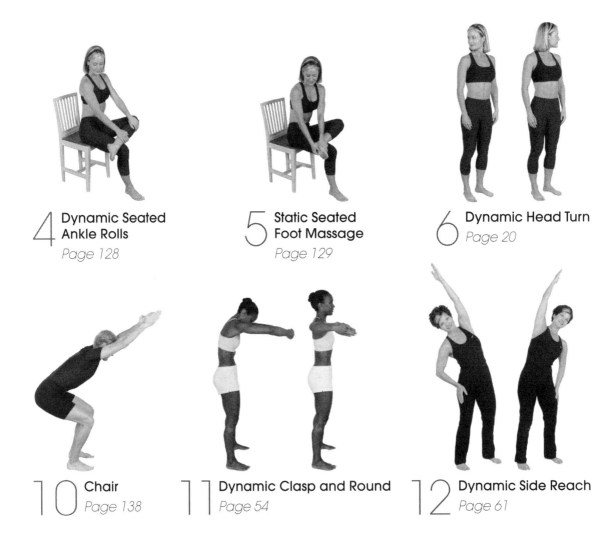

4 Dynamic Seated Ankle Rolls
Page 128

5 Static Seated Foot Massage
Page 129

6 Dynamic Head Turn
Page 20

10 Chair
Page 138

11 Dynamic Clasp and Round
Page 54

12 Dynamic Side Reach
Page 61

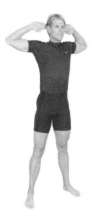

Static Chest Expansion
Page 50

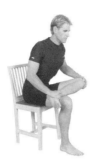

2 **Static Seated Figure 4 (on chair)**
Page 72

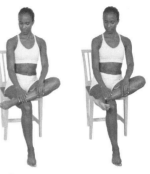

3 **Dynamic Seated Toe Flex and Point**
Page 130

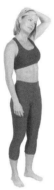

7 **Static Head Tilt**
Page 16

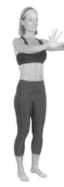

8 **Dynamic Web Hands**
Page 46

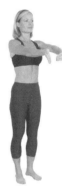

9 **Dynamic Wrist Rolls**
Page 42

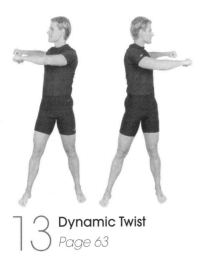

13 **Dynamic Twist**
Page 63

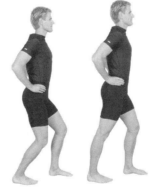

14 **Dynamic Bent-Knee Heel Press**
Page 121

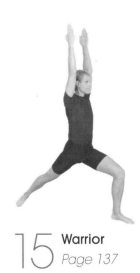

15 **Warrior**
Page 137

EVENING STRETCH ROUTINE

Approximate time: 10 minutes

This routine starts you on your feet and finishes you on the floor. I recommend it for right before you go to bed. It's a perfect way to end your day. The stretches focus on the areas most commonly tight at the end of the day. You'll feel relaxed and will get a better night's sleep.

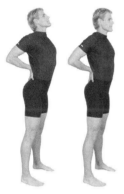

1 **Dynamic Arch**
Page 68

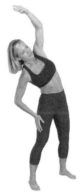

2 **Static Side Reach**
Page 59

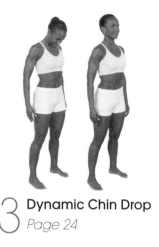

3 **Dynamic Chin Drop**
Page 24

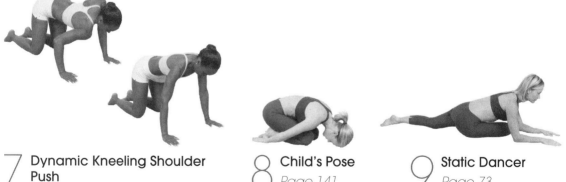

7 **Dynamic Kneeling Shoulder Push**
Page 28

8 **Child's Pose**
Page 141

9 **Static Dancer**
Page 73

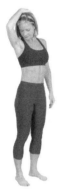

4 **Static Diagonal Head Tilt**
Page 17

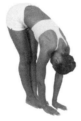

5 **Forward Bend**
Page 142

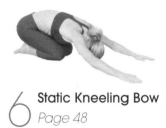

6 **Static Kneeling Bow**
Page 48

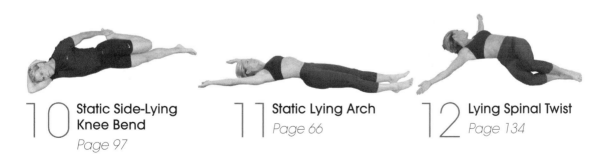

10 **Static Side-Lying Knee Bend**
Page 97

11 **Static Lying Arch**
Page 66

12 **Lying Spinal Twist**
Page 134

HEALTHY BACK ROUTINE

Approximate time: 10 minutes

This routine strengthens and stretches the most important muscles in your trunk and core. You'll have a healthier back and improved posture. If you have chronic back pain, please consult your physician before attempting this routine because some of the stretches are challenging. You'll begin standing, then do some stretches from a chair, and then from a seated position on the floor. This is a valuable sequence you can do anytime during the day or in conjunction with any of the other routines.

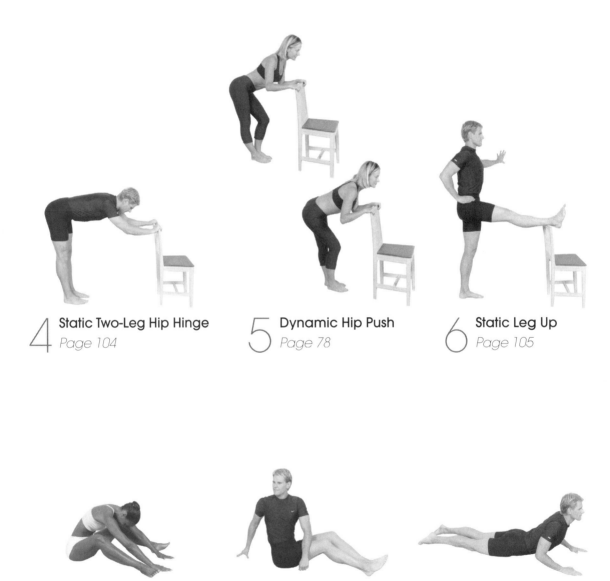

4 Static Two-Leg Hip Hinge
Page 104

5 Dynamic Hip Push
Page 78

6 Static Leg Up
Page 105

10 Static Seated Forward Bend
Page 55

11 Static Seated Twist
Page 62

12 Static Cobra
Page 64

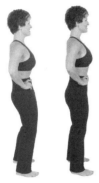
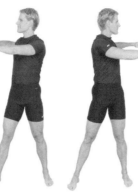
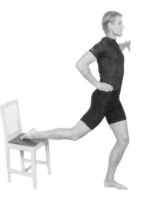

1 Dynamic Pelvic Tilt
Page 57

2 Dynamic Twist
Page 63

3 Static Anchored Lunge
Page 83

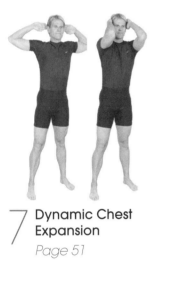
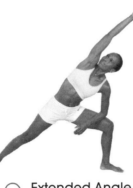
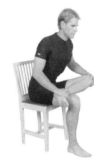

7 Dynamic Chest Expansion
Page 51

8 Extended Angle
Page 136

9 Static Seated Figure 4 (on chair)
Page 72

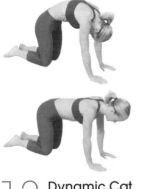
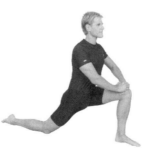
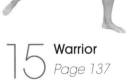

13 Dynamic Cat
Page 58

14 Static Kneeling Runner's Lunge
Page 82

15 Warrior
Page 137

STRESS-FREE NECK AND SHOULDERS ROUTINE

Approximate time: 5 minutes

This routine is perfect if you experience a tight neck or carry your stress in your shoulder area. It's a simple routine that takes only five minutes and can be done right at your desk during the day. When you do this routine, you'll notice your shoulders and neck immediately feel more relaxed, which usually makes it easier to concentrate. Do this routine as often as you like, whenever you need a quick break or feel yourself slouching at your desk.

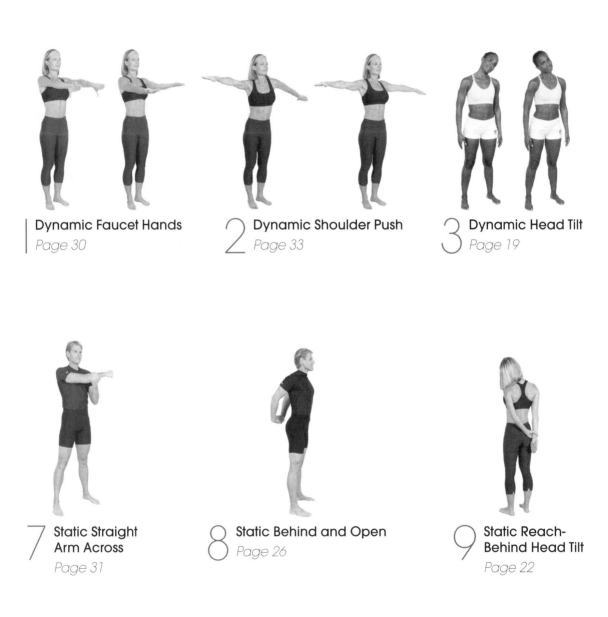

1 Dynamic Faucet Hands
Page 30

2 Dynamic Shoulder Push
Page 33

3 Dynamic Head Tilt
Page 19

7 Static Straight Arm Across
Page 31

8 Static Behind and Open
Page 26

9 Static Reach-Behind Head Tilt
Page 22

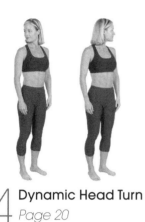

4 **Dynamic Head Turn**
Page 20

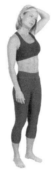
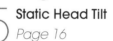

5 **Static Head Tilt**
Page 16

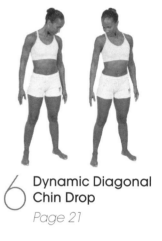

6 **Dynamic Diagonal Chin Drop**
Page 21

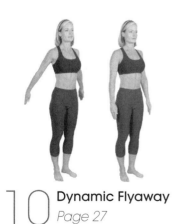

10 **Dynamic Flyaway**
Page 27

UPPER BODY STRETCH ROUTINE

Approximate time: 10 minutes

This routine focuses on the muscles above the waist and hip. Try this routine if you use your upper body a lot during the day, or if you have done an activity that stresses the upper body, such as snow shoveling, painting, or washing the car.

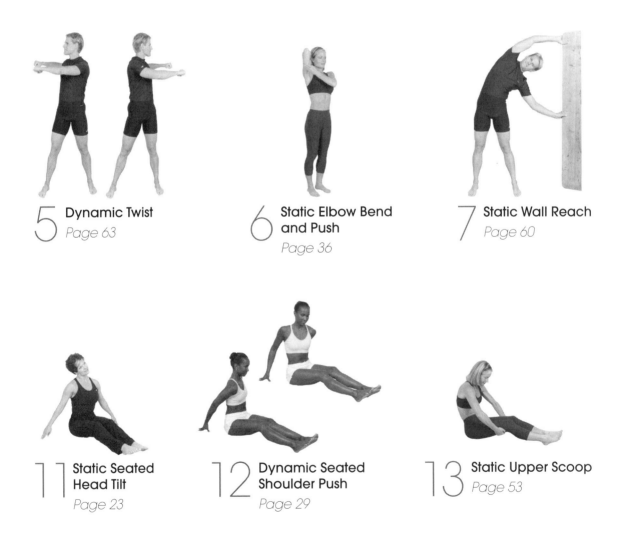

5 **Dynamic Twist**
Page 63

6 **Static Elbow Bend and Push**
Page 36

7 **Static Wall Reach**
Page 60

11 **Static Seated Head Tilt**
Page 23

12 **Dynamic Seated Shoulder Push**
Page 29

13 **Static Upper Scoop**
Page 53

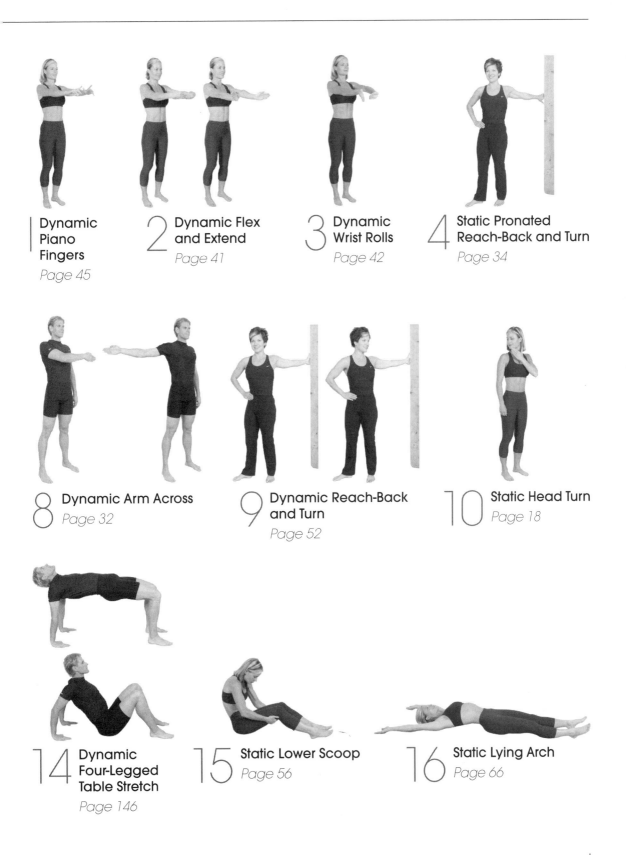

1. Dynamic Piano Fingers
Page 45

2. Dynamic Flex and Extend
Page 41

3. Dynamic Wrist Rolls
Page 42

4. Static Pronated Reach-Back and Turn
Page 34

8. Dynamic Arm Across
Page 32

9. Dynamic Reach-Back and Turn
Page 52

10. Static Head Turn
Page 18

14. Dynamic Four-Legged Table Stretch
Page 146

15. Static Lower Scoop
Page 56

16. Static Lying Arch
Page 66

LOWER BODY STRETCH ROUTINE

Approximate time: 12 minutes

This routine is for the muscles below the waist and hip. Try this one if you use your lower body a lot during the day, or if you have done an activity that stresses the lower body, such as climbing stairs, playing chase, or hiking.

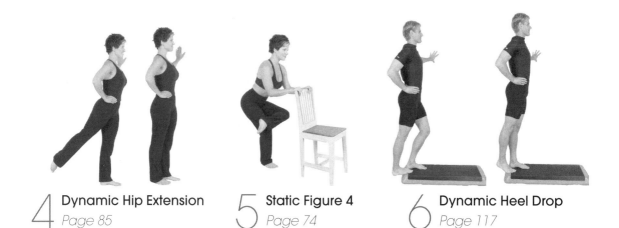

4 **Dynamic Hip Extension**
Page 85

5 **Static Figure 4**
Page 74

6 **Dynamic Heel Drop**
Page 117

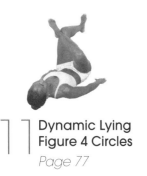

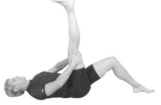

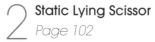

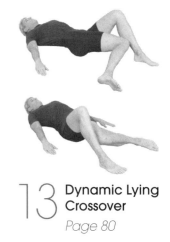

11 **Dynamic Lying Figure 4 Circles**
Page 77

12 **Static Lying Scissor**
Page 102

13 **Dynamic Lying Crossover**
Page 80

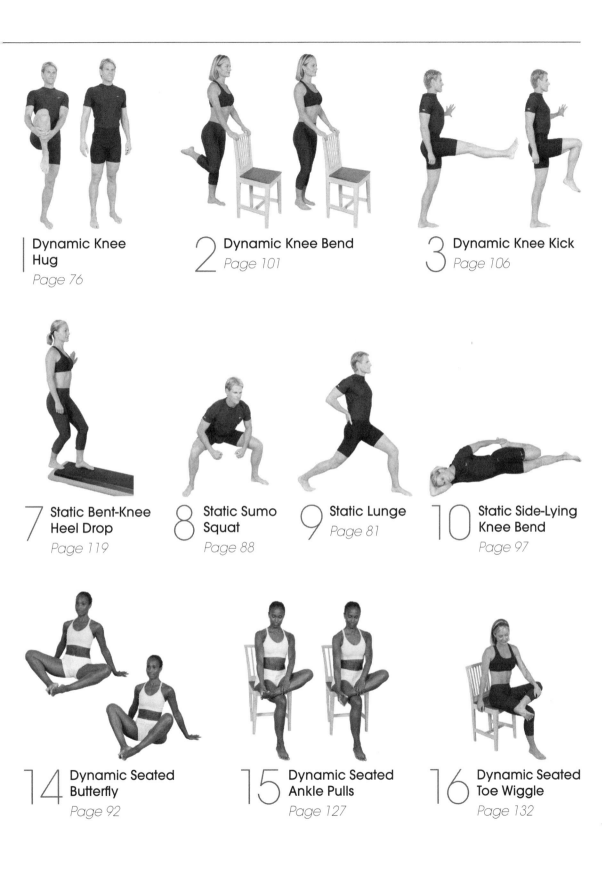

1 Dynamic Knee Hug
Page 76

2 Dynamic Knee Bend
Page 101

3 Dynamic Knee Kick
Page 106

7 Static Bent-Knee Heel Drop
Page 119

8 Static Sumo Squat
Page 88

9 Static Lunge
Page 81

10 Static Side-Lying Knee Bend
Page 97

14 Dynamic Seated Butterfly
Page 92

15 Dynamic Seated Ankle Pulls
Page 127

16 Dynamic Seated Toe Wiggle
Page 132

BEND, REACH, AND PLAY ROUTINE

Approximate time: 5 to 15 minutes

This routine makes it easier for you to bend, reach, and play. If you want to improve your ability to get around, play with your kids, or just do simple everyday tasks such as gardening or washing the car, this is a good routine for you. This is my favorite sequence because it's inspired by the sun salutation in yoga and can be done just about anywhere or anytime. You can do the sequence just once or, ideally, repeat it three to five times, which of course takes longer but is well worth it. You might be surprised how such a simple routine can make you feel so much better.

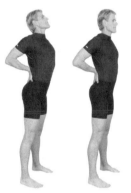

1 **Dynamic Arch**
Page 68

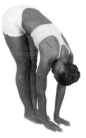

2 **Forward Bend**
Page 142

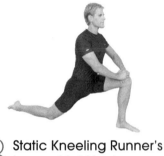

3 **Static Kneeling Runner's Lunge (right leg)**
Page 82

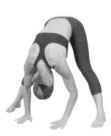

7 **Fan**
Page 144

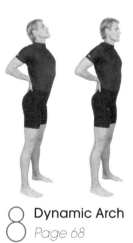

8 **Dynamic Arch**
Page 68

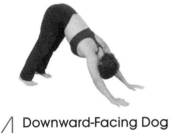

4 **Downward-Facing Dog**
Page 139

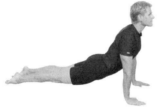

5 **Upward-Facing Dog**
Page 140

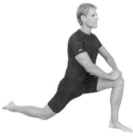

6 **Static Kneeling Runner's Lunge (left leg)**
Page 82

INDEX

Note: The italicized *f* following a page number denotes a figure on that page. The italicized *ff* following a page number denotes multiple figures on that page.

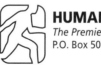